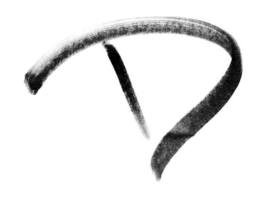

The Gentle Greeting

An Obstetrician's Guide

to Planning a Loving Pregnancy

and Birth Experience

Ronald L. Cole, M.D.

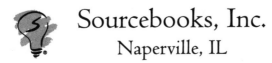

Sourcebooks, Inc.
Naperville, IL

Published by Sourcebooks, Inc.
P.O. Box 372, Naperville, IL 60566
630-961-3900
Fax: 630-961-2168

This publication is designed to provide accurate and authoritative information in regard to the subject matter covered. It is sold with the understanding that the publisher is not engaged in rendering legal, accounting, or other professional service. If legal advice or other expert assistance is required, the services of a competent professional person should be sought.

From a Declaration of Principles Jointly Adopted by a Committee of the American Bar Association and a Committee of Publishers and Associations

Publisher's Note
It is our intention that the information in this book be used solely under the guidance and supervision of a qualified health professional. Diligent efforts have been made to assure the accuracy and safety of this information for a general audience. Nonetheless, different individuals require different health care needs. This book is not intended to provide medical advice, nor is it to be used as a substitute for advice from your own physician. The information is presented without guarantees from the author and publisher, who disclaim all liability or responsibility in connection with any mishaps or damage caused, or alleged to be caused, directly or indirectly, by the information contained in this book.

Library of Congress Cataloging-in-Publication Data
Cole, Ronald L.
     The gentle greeting: an obstetrician's guide to planning a loving pregnancy and birth experience / Ronald L. Cole.
          p.   cm.
     Includes index.
     ISBN 1-57071-325-1 (alk. paper)
     1. Prenatal care—Popular works.   2. Prenatal influencing—Popular works.
3. Pregnancy.   4. Childbirth.   5. Physician and Patient.
I. Title.
RG525.C683   1998
618.2—dc21
                                                                    98-10357
                                                                    CIP

Printed and bound in the United States of America
10   9   8   7   6   5   4   3   2   1

To
Ed and Mary Cole
Loving Parents
who gave their heart, soul, and energy
to their three children
Carey
Ron
Marcia

Contents

Part II   *Designing a Gentle Birth*

Part III   Labor, Delivery, and Postnatal Care

Acknowledgments

IT HAS TAKEN many years of study and experience to prepare for and then actually write this book. In the course of this spiritual journey, I have been influenced and supported by many people who I would like to acknowledge and thank.

I would first like to acknowledge the Oneness of Mother Nature, the Universe, the inherent Love, Perfection, and Beauty of which she is composed, and the wonderful spiritual Truth, which is available simply for the asking.

Reverend Beverly Burdick-Carey has been a special source of truth and enlightenment to me for many years.

I would like to thank the great labor and delivery nurses I have worked with, particularly those who bring a loving attitude in the labor and delivery room. I have always felt that they are worth their weight in gold, and I appreciate their support and contribution to my evolution over the years. A special thanks goes to Marcy Hammons, my office nurse and previous labor and delivery nurse, and to Glinda Craig, my office manager, for their efforts and belief in what I am trying to achieve, starting from the "early years."

A special thanks to BayCoast Hospital for their support in helping bring to reality many needed changes in the birth experience.

I would like to acknowledge the Association for Pre- and Perinatal Psychology and Health, its founder, Thomas Verny, M.D., its current president, David Chamberlain, Ph.D., and all of its members, who are dedicated to improving the ultimate first impression.

I would like to acknowledge the efforts of Katharine Bernard whose talents as an editor and enlightened thinker helped greatly in creating the finished book. I would also like to thank both The Hart Agency and Sourcebooks, Inc., for their belief in me and my work as well as their faith in making this first of many works become a reality.

I have had invaluable help and support from my family, friends, evolved protectors and teachers, and many other sources for which I am indeed thankful. I could not have come this far in my physical and spiritual journey without the love and support I have received from a myriad of sources. May the journey honor the love and perfection of the universe, particularly our small part in it.

Credit goes to you, the reader, to all parents and families desiring a loving birth experience, and all of the many medical and non-medical people who have dedicated time and effort to improving the pregnancy and birth experience. Only through combined effort will we create the ultimate birth experience. Hold fast to your convictions, and change will come.

Finally, I would like to acknowledge and thank all of the parents and babies whose births I have been privileged to play a part in.

Introduction

BIRTH—we have all experienced it first-hand, and many of us have also participated in or witnessed the birth of loved ones. Babies are born every hour of every day. Most of us take the perpetuation of life for granted and do not appreciate the complicated, unique miracle of birth until it comes into our own lives.

If you are reading this book, your life has probably been touched by the prospect of new life. As an obstetrician/gynecologist, I have been privileged to witness the development and finally the birth of many babies. It is always similar and yet ever unique, just as we are. Birth is, after all, our first impression of life.

But, my experience has also left me feeling that a traditional hospital delivery falls short of the gentle, loving welcome new life deserves. Traditional medicine gets the job done as safely as possible but needs to be lovingly humanized both for the parents and for the baby.

My purpose in writing this book is to make people aware of the possibilities, the availability, and the advantages of a holistic approach to pregnancy and a more gentle, loving, family-oriented hospital birth.

I did not start out on this mission. I took the long way around to get where I am today, but I arrived here, in part, because of births in my own experience.

Three births that have personally touched my life's experience help to illustrate the wide variety that birth experiences can take and some of the reasons I have come to have such strong views on childbirth.

My own birth experience, often related to me by my beloved father, occurred over fifty years ago. As he told it, an intern was watching over the labor and delivery, and my father overheard him tell the nurse to double up on Pitocin (a medication that induces contractions) because he wanted to deliver the baby himself. Very soon, my father could tell from my mother's reactions that I was ready to arrive and went running for the nurse, calling, "My wife is ready to have the baby, and the doctor isn't here!" Soon, Dr. Taylor came running in and proceeded to deliver me. According to my father, once the delivery was completed, the doctor also gave the intern a piece of his mind. So, I made a swift entry into the world, having received a medical "kick in the pants!"

The next birth I personally experienced was the birth of my first son, Ted Edward Cole. I was in the Army in Salt Lake City, Utah. There were no obstetrical services available on the base, so we chose a civilian obstetrician. This was in 1968, and I had certainly never heard of "natural childbirth." By chance, we found an obstetrician who was ahead of his time and open to the idea of allowing "natural" and family-inclusive childbirth. When my wife went into labor, I was not only allowed to be with her during labor as well as the delivery, but I was allowed to photograph the entire event!

It was a joyful and moving event for our family, resulting in our beautiful, healthy baby. I had no idea at the time that many years later,

I would be working to encourage and standardize this family approach to childbirth.

In sharp contrast to those two birth experiences was the birth of my second son, Kent James Cole. I was then out of the Army, had fulfilled my ROTC commitment, and was embarking on an engineering career. Having had such a wonderful experience with the birth of our first child, I wanted to find a physician who would allow me to be in the delivery room. The first physician we interviewed was somewhat hesitant. Having recently delivered a baby with a severe birth defect, he was not comfortable with the idea and asked us, "What if a similar birth occurred?"

We found another physician who, somewhat reluctantly, agreed to let me be in the delivery room. Near the time of delivery, it was discovered that Kent was in the breech (bottom first) position. Our physician called another doctor in to assist him, and I was asked to leave the delivery room. I had no idea how this delivery would dramatically change my life forever and even contribute to a major career change.

Everything seemed to be okay. The delivery went well, and I felt good about that. However, not long after that, they brought Kent out wrapped in a blanket. The doctor said, "It's a boy." Then he added that there was a little problem with his back, and he would have to stay in the hospital a little longer and might require surgery.

I asked what the problem was. The physician said that Kent appeared to have a condition called spina bifida.

"Spina what?" I asked.

I had no idea what spina bifida was and no indication of its severity. My wife and I could only look at Kent and wonder what was going on. They sent for a specialist.

Ironically, spina bifida or "open spine" was the birth defect the first doctor we interviewed referred to. In fact, due to spending a great deal of time at the hospital with Kent, we became well-acquainted with Angela, the baby with this birth defect whom that doctor had delivered, and her parents, Buddy and Tricia.

A few hours later, the neurosurgeon came to talk with us. He dropped quite a bombshell. Instead of "a little problem," he was talking about surgeries, possible paralysis, and a wheelchair existence. We were caught completely off guard. To say the least, no tact was used; it felt like being hit with a 2x4! The neurosurgeon then added that they would soon take Kent into surgery to close the defect on his back.

At six hours old, Kent was wheeled into surgery for the first of what turned out to be about twenty-seven surgeries over the next number of years. We were dazed and uncertain, but realizing the need for the surgery, we proceeded without delay, not fully knowing the outcome. I tried to comfort my wife. We could only just begin to realize that our baby had a permanent, significant birth defect.

During the course of life, a specific event can cause us to review the path we are on and even motivate us to change in midstream. Sometimes, these changes are small or subtle. Other times, this shift can be the beginning of something that moves us in the direction of our heart and soul's calling.

September 29, 1969, the beginning of Kent's life, was also a day that would factor into a major life change for me. I began to fully realize the potential of knowledge, hope, love, and a positive attitude.

Soon after Kent's birth, I was contacted by the local Spina Bifida Association and received information and support on Kent's condition. I became convinced that I could help Kent conquer the crippling handicap. In 1971, about a year and a half after Kent's birth, I became president of the Association. This position gave me the opportunity to share with others the fact that hope and love are the strongest medicines you can give to yourself and your child when dealing with what seems to be an insurmountable liability. This also led me, along with others, to form the Spina Bifida Association of America.

The ability to realize what is in your control and what is beyond it is truly liberating. I couldn't control the fact that my son had been born with a birth defect, but I could take full and active control over teaching my son to meet and overcome the daily challenges of growing up, thus enabling him to mature and lead a productive and satisfying life. The knowledge I had gained, the hope in my heart, the love for my child and a positive attitude kept me going.

Kent is now twenty-eight years old and uses a wheelchair. He has been through a lot and has developed many strengths. He has been involved with Wheel Chair Olympics and weightlifting and is now training to become a veterinarian technician.

These three birth experiences that have played important roles in my life demonstrate that you never know exactly what to expect. Introspection caused me to recognize and acknowledge an inner calling that I had turned away from at the end of high school. I squelched this pure and real desire to become a physician, because I was afraid I could not achieve the goal. I went on to become a civil engineer instead. In the years to follow, I received my Master of Science in engineering and pursued an engineering career.

However, in the midst of Kent's medical trials and my continued involvement with the medical profession, I became dissatisfied with my engineering career. An inner calling to the medical field resurfaced. This time, I decided to meet the challenge, but there was now much to do to achieve my dream of being a doctor.

First, I had to complete two years of premed studies at night school to meet admission requirements. This accomplished, I applied and was accepted to medical school at my *alma mater*, the University of Missouri.

I resigned my position at Exxon Chemical Co., sold our family home, and with my wife and two children—one with major medical needs—moved to Columbia, Missouri.

My interest was in general surgery, and I clearly remember late in my second year of medical school assuredly stating that obstetrics and gynecology was "the *last* specialty I would want." Yet, for reasons I did not fully understand for years, I ended up choosing OB/GYN as my specialty.

Once in private practice, my approach to medicine was traditional. During this period, however, I developed a deep interest in the spiritual aspects of life and began reading, studying, and researching. I began to realize the potential of approaching pregnancy and birth holistically, without separating the physical from the mental and spiritual.

The creation of a human being involves the development of the complex human body, a process we do not yet fully understand. Many of us also believe that this body is joined by the spirit or soul, an aspect that is even more mysterious. It occurred to me that this side of humanity was not even recognized in the traditional medical birthing process.

Studying the pioneering work of others, combined with my own experience, I became convinced that health care providers could greatly expand and improve birth and healing by treating the whole person. This holistic approach does not in any way disregard medical science. We should be grateful for the advances and contributions made by the medical profession and the profound effect they have had on our health and well-being. That said, we must also recognize that improvements and advances in the way physicians practice medicine will ultimately benefit us all.

Because of my desire to combine the physical and nonphysical aspects of pregnancy and childbirth, I started researching and applying techniques to enhance the traditional experience without compromising safe obstetrical principles. Since the great majority of obstetrical experiences are normal, medically uneventful, healthy events, there is considerable room for flexibility.

I am sure most of my professional colleagues would say that early and good prenatal care and diet are the most important factors in achieving a healthy birth outcome. I fully agree that these are very important, but I have also come to realize that the core factor in achieving a good obstetrical outcome is simply creating a positive, loving attitude and atmosphere around the conception and pregnancy.

Unfortunately, principles of a nonphysical or spiritual nature are difficult to prove and are easily dismissed. They are certainly not included in formal academic training before or during medical school or residency, although this is slowly starting to change.

I believe love is the all-powerful force that drives the universe, and this force can be actively used to help achieve any positive goal, including a good obstetrical outcome. In my practice, I am a strong advocate for good, up-to-date obstetrics. But I also believe that while good obstetrics come first, the birthing experience can be enhanced by recognizing the higher spiritual aspects surrounding pregnancy, birth, and the creation of life.

Once I saw that treating pregnancy and birth holistically had a positive affect on both parents and newborns, I saw the need to share this approach. Anticipated criticism was soon directed toward some of my delivery practices, such as talking to the unborn child, dimming lights in the delivery room, playing music, involving family members, directing love and consideration to the unborn/newborn child, and encouraging bonding by having the baby stay with the parents rather than being taken immediately to the nursery. While none of these practices is in any way medically dangerous or even radical, they still met with much resistance and criticism from the medical community.

I continued to search for and incorporate new ways to make pregnancy and birth as gentle and loving as possible. In the beginning, use of whirlpool baths for laboring mothers was scoffed at, but after statistics showed that there was no increase of infection for the laboring mother, the use of a properly maintained whirlpool for labor became common and is now a standard available feature in many hospitals. Once the record of my deliveries proved to be as good as or better than those practicing "traditional" deliveries, the initial uproar and criticism from my colleagues regarding my approach began to die down. Moreover, I began to see that the medical community was responding more readily to consumer demand. When enough parents believe in and demand gentle birthing practices, the medical profession will stand up and take notice.

Over the last twelve years, I have greatly expanded my understanding of combining spiritual and medical principles. My belief that the unborn child has his or her own soul from or before the moment of conception has never wavered.

My belief that the soul continues to exist in a spiritual plane stems from a common thread that runs through many of the world's religions. If you believe in a continuum of life after death, then you must consider from whence you came before birth! Where did your individual soul come from? Your answer may come from religious beliefs or from your own personal contemplation or study. If you believe the human spirit exists before birth, then you can appreciate the value and importance of "talking" to the unborn child. This early communication with the child has been deeply meaningful to many prospective parents and a boon during many deliveries.

Over time, I have chosen a subtle approach to convey the full integration of physical, mental, and spiritual aspects of pregnancy and birth.

My goal in writing this book is to help make the birth experience what most parents hope it will be: a medically safe, loving, family celebration that can be remembered as one of the most extraordinary events of their lives. Over the years, I have changed from a traditional obstetrician/gynecologist to one who has learned and demonstrated that the birth experience is the ultimate first expression of love. My hope is that sharing what I have learned helps you to understand that the birth experience can and should be for, about, and tailored— within the bounds of sound medicine—to the desires of each family. Furthermore, there are several safe, alternative additions that can greatly enhance the birth experience. I also wish to offer support to parents who want an individualized birth experience, and I urge them to seek out a physician who shares their desires. It is your body, your baby, your birth experience.

Birth is the ultimate first impression of life, and love is the most powerful and useful source of energy. You can make your pregnancy and birth experience reflect all of the positive aspects of these simple principles. In turn, we can all continue to learn and incorporate a more thorough understanding of the synergy between spiritual and medical principles to allow life and its beginning to be enlightening.

—Ronald L. Cole, M.D.

A Special Note to Physicians

I totally support the obstetrical techniques taught in medical school and residency. I use the excellent training I received in my practice every day. But, I urge "traditional" physicians to open up their own hearts and minds and add loving attitudes and principles to their practice of obstetrics.

I have learned through many years of experience that traditional medicine has a difficult time accepting nontraditional thinking, particularly if it cannot be evaluated by a double-blind, cross-over statistical study. Any physician willing to give this "dose of love" an honest chance will be rewarded. The power of true love from the heart can add to any endeavor. Remember, love is infectious!

Part I

Pregnancy Planning and Prenatal Care

1

Birth

The Ultimate First Impression

PICTURE YOURSELF as a first time visitor to a foreign country, a little apprehensive because you do not know the language and you have never met your awaiting relatives. After a comfortable flight, you enter an extremely crowded airport where everyone is pushing, shoving, and squeezing you. The airport authorities seem preoccupied, unfriendly, and pay you little attention. Then a security guard grabs you and takes you into a small, cold, bright room. First they search you, then they take you to another room where they run medical tests on you without any explanation or reassurance. After being poked and prodded, you are forced to take a bath. Finally, after several hours, you are released from your room and taken to meet your family.

Not a very loving or welcoming reception and certainly not one you would like to repeat or would soon forget. Sadly, it is analogous to the first greeting most babies receive! We all know the deep and long-lasting effect of a first impression. What impression could be more important than our very first experience in this world!

Many people, physicians and parents alike, wonder why we should be so concerned about making an effort to give the newborn child a more gentle and loving first impression. Supposedly, the infant is not aware enough to know what's taking place at birth. Nothing could be further from the truth! There is a large body of research and literature available today to support the idea that we come into this life with an awareness of the feelings and emotions around us. Research also shows that we retain a detailed but subconscious memory of our birth experience, which can influence us throughout our entire lives.

My own experience with expectant parents and in the birthing room has made me keenly aware of the spirit within the unborn and newborn child. Unfortunately, the rather rigid ideas taught at our medical schools and in our residency programs often result in inflexible physicians, focused narrowly on the physical world, who feel that only they know what is best for the patient.

For the first few years of my career as an OB/GYN, I, too, diligently practiced the physical/medical aspects of obstetrics as I was taught in medical school. Pregnancies were achieved and monitored, and babies were born. I was accomplishing my mission. But, my daily involvement with the natural wonder of birth and a long-time study of the spiritual aspects of life slowly led me to realize that much was missing from my knowledge and in my practice of birth and healing.

Observations made within my practice combined with further study and research led me to realize that by focusing on the medical/technical/physical aspects of the birth process, those of us in the medical community were either ignoring or obscuring the importance of the emotional and spiritual aspects surrounding conception, pregnancy, and birth.

With this realization, I began taking a more holistic approach to my practice, recognizing the importance and the inseparability of the physical, mental, emotional, and spiritual components within each conception, pregnancy, and birth. An awareness of the soul is indispensible to the best practice of medicine. Opening my mind as well as my eyes to new possibilities has explained many mysteries that the traditional medical/physical beliefs cannot.

I firmly believe that following sound obstetrical practice is always the number one priority, particularly if complications occur. However, keep in mind that with any normal pregnancy, there is ample room for individualizing and enhancing the birth experience. During the years since I changed my approach, I have been amazed and delighted by many of the birth experiences my patients have created and the effect they have had on the babies themselves.

The purpose of this book is not to replace the current techniques and practices of obstetrics, but to promote a greater understanding of all aspects of prenatal life and birth in order to help each expectant family appreciate their options for a deeply fulfilling pregnancy and a gentle (for mother *and* baby), personalized, family-oriented birth experience. I offer the insights I have gained in my life and my practice with the hope that each family will use them in their own way, taking responsibility for creating their own "right" circumstances and feeling pride in their efforts and choices.

The three keys to a good birth experience are education, preparation, and a positive attitude. Education and preparation take time and effort on behalf of both the family and the physician. The family needs to learn about pregnancy—the physical changes that both mother and baby undergo—and explore the world of the unborn. The parents also need to research their birthing options to be sure they have the most satisfying and fulfilling delivery possible.

The obstetrician needs to encourage questions, provide sound and sensitive answers, explain, inform, and refer expectant families to helpful, informative materials, such as handouts, books, videos, and Lamaze and other childbirth classes.

The handouts I use and books I refer expectant parents to cover practice logistics, labor guides, sibling preparation, and a variety of material on the physical development and spiritual aspects of the unborn child, as well as birthing alternatives. With the cooperation of my patients, I have produced several videotapes to illustrate loving, positive, family-oriented childbirth. I strongly recommend Lamaze and childbirth education classes. They are helpful, informative, and supportive, especially for first births. I make all of these materials available to my patients, but it is up to them to take full advantage of them.

Getting Started

There is a fascinating wealth of information available to parents-to-be. The following books will get you started.

To learn more about the prebirth experience of the child, look for *The Secret Life of the Unborn Child,* by Thomas Verny, M.D., and *Life before Life,* by Helen Wambach, Ph.D.

Ideal Birth, by Sondra Ray, R.N., gives an overview of gentle birthing alternatives.

To learn more about the impact of the birth experience, *Babies Remember Birth*, by David Chamberlain, Ph.D., is an excellent start.

One of my primary motivations in writing this book is to convey my conviction that every pregnancy is directly influenced by attitudes, emotions, and thoughts. To begin with, feeling receptive to life can actually help achieve a pregnancy. Further, attitudes, emotions, and thoughts are often evident throughout the pregnancy and even in the newborn.

The atmosphere surrounding a pregnancy is created by the *expectant mother's* attitudes, beliefs, self-image, thoughts, and actions, as well as by all of the other people who are close to the mother, most importantly, the father. Positive, loving thoughts and attitudes help generate the same in pregnancy, delivery, and life. The emotional atmosphere within the family—be it tranquil, stimulating, tense, or turbulent—has a significant impact on the unborn child. This external atmosphere surrounding the mother, combined with the mother's internal attitudes, emotions, and thoughts, is reflected throughout the progress of the pregnancy, the delivery, and the birth outcome.

Attitude so influences each birth experience that I am able to fairly accurately predict what a couple's experience will be by their questions, family participation, and interest in learning. It is a great joy to have the opportunity to work with prospective parents who are loving and involved. The process as well as the outcome of such pregnancies and deliveries is a beautiful tribute to the human spirit.

Thus, a good birth experience depends to a great extent on the attitudes as well as the actions of the entire family. Positive thoughts and actions build upon themselves. Feeling positive and finding inner peace can be the most productive step you can take during pregnancy for yourself and your unborn child. However, there are a number of steps that the new mother and father can take to see that the newest member has a wonderful first impression. They will be fully explored throughout this book, but here is an overview.

- Practice active family planning so that your pregnancy is expected. This gives the most positive start to any pregnancy.

- Make the pregnancy a family affair, involving all family members. This begins the bonding process and eases the newborn's transition into the family.

- Commit to making the effort that will ensure the best and most fulfilling and enjoyable outcome.

- Contemplate and communicate how you, as a family, want your birth experience to be orchestrated.

- Recognize that communication with your unborn child can start right away. Those around the unborn child should talk to him/her in a loving, intelligent way. Read stories, sing songs, and play pleasant music for the new baby.

- Take care of your body during pregnancy: eat sensibly, exercise, and rest. Make it a priority to break detrimental habits—smoking, drinking alcohol, and drug consumption—before you get pregnant.

- Find a qualified obstetrician who is willing to listen to your desires, personalize the birth and prenatal experiences, encourage family involvement, and show care and empathy for the child and family.

- Do not be afraid to ask questions. Your obstetrician should encourage questions, not avoid them. If the physician does not explain medical information so that you can understand it, the fault is with the physician, not you.

- Be aware that a common reason given by many obstetricians for not using more innovative techniques (whirlpool, dim lights, children present, providing flexibility to the laboring mother, etc.) is that they are risky. These doctors' medical education and lack of personal experience with innovative techniques may lead them to believe that such innovations are unsafe. However, these methods have been used safely for years and have enhanced many birth experiences.

- When you know what kind of delivery you want, stick to your convictions. Remember, it is your birth experience, not the obstetrician's. If you cannot see eye-to-eye, change doctors. When you find your ideal obstetrician, let your friends know about it.

• Visit the labor and delivery unit at the hospital where your obstetrician delivers. Talk to the nurses. You can learn a lot from them about the philosophies and techniques of the various doctors.

• Create your own emotional environment through visualization, meditation, and positive thinking. Positive attitudes and thoughts create positive, joyful experiences. Look forward to them.

• Let go of your preconceived notions and the well-intentioned advice from others concerning labor and delivery. Do not program yourself to expect pain.

One of the most meaningful events in a couple's life is the birth of their child. Moreover, the time and energy spent by parents to raise a child is a significant part of their lives. Considering this, it makes perfect sense that the love and extra effort put into the birth experience will pay tremendous dividends to all those involved. Do not settle for a second-rate birth experience or your doctor's "routine" delivery. Take responsibility for creating a unique and loving, as well as medically safe, ultimate first impression. Both the parents and the child deserve the best birth experience possible.

Now, let's concentrate on bringing your new life into the world. As we proceed with the specifics of creating your own personal birth experience, I will point out how to apply this holistic viewpoint, starting with preconception planning and proceeding through to the gentle birth of your child.

2

Pregnancy Planning

Welcome New Life

MANY COUPLES first consult me when they are ready to have a child. I am always happy to see couples at this stage, because preconception planning allows prospective parents to begin their physical and medical preparation, as well as their spiritual and emotional preparation, at the outset. If you start your pregnancy in good health physically, mentally, emotionally, and spiritually, it will greatly enhance your pregnancy and birth experience.

Pregnancy planning and preparation begins with the basic relationship between the future mother and father. A loving relationship provides a receptive attitude, which is "fertile ground" for bringing new life into this world. The best start on any pregnancy will be achieved within the environment of a close, loving relationship and the shared desire to bring new life into the world.

Along with a stable, loving relationship, the smoothest transition into pregnancy occurs when it is planned. Having a baby is a major life change and commitment. The desire to have a baby and feeling ready to have a child helps couples anticipate and cope with the ensuing changes. When a pregnancy is planned and desired, it has a positive "jump start" because the couple's thoughts, emotions, and actions are already moving in the direction of becoming parents.

Pregnancy planning should also be practical. It costs a lot of money to have and raise a child. If a couple does not realistically evaluate their financial situation before they have a child, the added costs can cause considerable stress on the household. Today's cost of living and society's material expectations have forced many women out of the home, into the workplace, and away from their children. A thoughtful couple will carefully examine their priorities in order to bring their baby into the best possible situation for all.

Unplanned Pregnancies

Probably more than 50 percent of pregnancies are not consciously planned. In my experience, couples often find that after the initial shock wears off and the idea sinks in, they accept the pregnancy, and their involvement and excitement begin to grow. Unfortunately, some couples may feel guilty about their initial resentment or negative feelings toward the pregnancy. When this happens, I try to reassure the couple that they have done nothing wrong; they were only responding to an unexpected event. I urge such couples to evaluate their true feelings in order to release negativity and replace it with the rapidly building positive emotions they are experiencing.

The most common reason given for an unplanned pregnancy is that proper birth control methods were not used. Women who are certain they don't want to become pregnant make it their business to take the necessary steps to greatly reduce their chances of getting pregnant. While some women do become pregnant while using birth control, this accounts for only about 2 percent of pregnancies.

The conscious mind, the realm of the brain we best understand, accounts for only 15 percent of the human mind. The unconscious mind, accounting for the remaining 85 percent, remains largely mysterious, but we know it is a powerful force that influences our conscious actions. Consider the idea, then, that "accidental" pregnancies are not accidents at all but reflections of our unconscious desires and the influence of the unborn child.

To illustrate, I will relate an example I call "pregnancy against all odds." Nancy and Bob came to me during their third pregnancy. Their first child, Nancy told me, was conceived while she was taking birth control pills. Their second child was conceived while Nancy was on birth control pills and had an IUD in place. The baby I delivered, their third, was conceived despite a tubal ligation! After delivery, Nancy asked me to put an end to her childbearing. Since this woman was obviously determined, I agreed to remove her left and right fallopian tubes. Sure enough, one could plainly see the plastic clip was properly locked in place on each tube, physically and completely blocking them. There was no physical or medical explanation for her pregnancy, yet there was her child!

Infertility

What about couples who want to become pregnant and are trying to become pregnant but do not achieve pregnancy? According to obstetrical statistics, about 80 percent of couples who are using no birth control or who are actively trying to get pregnant achieve pregnancy within twelve months. An additional 10 percent will get pregnant over the following twelve months. That leaves, after two years, about 10 percent of couples who have not achieved pregnancy. These couples, like all patients, should be approached from a holistic standpoint, encompassing both the physical and nonphysical aspects of their concerns.

When should a couple seek infertility counseling? That decision should be left up to each couple and will vary from a few months to years. Initially, a complete medical history should be taken and a physical examination performed to see if there appears to be any medical reason for infertility. I also recommend several basic medical tests to evaluate the woman's ovulation and fallopian tubes and the man's ability to father children. I will frequently place the patient on a basal body temperature chart to help determine whether she is ovulating normally. If a medical problem, such as obstructed tubes, endometriosis, abnormal uterine anatomy, abnormal hormone levels, or chronic disease, is found, it should be evaluated and treated, if possible.

It has been my experience, and I am sure that of many OB/GYNs, that in a significant percent of infertility patients, no physical or medical reason can be found for the failure to become pregnant. The next step is to look for a nonphysical explanation. One nonphysical cause is the lack of true desire for a child—the unconscious at work again. Many people will say they want to have a child, but their hearts and minds are not really dedicated to it. Most of us have been brought up to believe that everyone is supposed to get married and have children. In reality, especially in today's society, it is perfectly okay to delay having children, to opt not to have children, or to not want additional children. I am convinced that if the mind and spirit do not want or are not really ready for pregnancy, they can prevent the body from getting pregnant by unconsciously affecting the immune system and the hormonal balance.

A few years back, Eileen and David, a couple in their late thirties/early forties came to see me. They had been to almost every infertility expert in the area, and had been through multiple tests, treatments, and even surgeries in their effort to become pregnant. Initially, we did a routine evaluation and even an outpatient surgery. Having done what we could medically, I again questioned their true desire to have a child. They thought for a while, discussed it, and came back with this response. "We have a pretty good life," David said. "We travel a lot in our RV and really enjoy it. Now that we have rethought it and talked it over, we realize that a baby would dramatically change the lifestyle we love, and we're not sure we want to give it up to have a child."

David and Eileen were caught up in their quest to have a baby, but their hearts were not dedicated to having a child. It took them a long time to realize what they really wanted because they had not reexamined their true desires along the way. Once they thought it out, considering their desires and not those of their families, they realized they did not want to alter the life they had come to love. They were finally able to give themselves permission to not have a baby.

Another nonphysical obstacle to pregnancy can be the guilt, negative feelings, or strong emotional issues surrounding past experiences, such as abortion(s) or unhappy childhood memories of abandonment, divorce, or physical or emotional abuse.

What would be the treatment for this kind of infertility? It has been my experience that simply talking to the patient and encouraging her to confront, work through, and resolve the negative emotions connected to such experiences can be therapeutic. It usually takes one-on-one, in-depth, gentle questioning to help the patient open up and reveal important past history. Some women may prefer to work with a psychologist, or religious or spiritual advisor; some prefer to work it out by themselves. In any case, the OB/GYN can help by encouraging patients to believe that they can have a happy and loving pregnancy.

Let's take the case of a patient I will call Linda. After appropriate questioning, she revealed a history of repeated child abuse she suffered by her father. The renewed memories obviously upset her, but we worked through it. Eventually, she discussed her guilt and fear. She particularly feared that the same thing could happen to a child she might bear, even though there was no current basis for that fear. As she described her husband's personality and her relationship with him, she began to realize that she was perpetuating her own unresolved past fears and that they were subconsciously interfering with her normal reproductive functions. Linda went home, feeling as if a burden had been lifted from her. She was ready for pregnancy. The fascinating part is that all it took was a change of attitude. It is so easy, yet so hard. As you may have guessed, Linda returned a few months later to confirm that she was, indeed, pregnant.

Laura presented a different aspect of this scenario. From the obstetrical history she gave, she had not had a previous pregnancy. However, during an office visit without her husband, she revealed that she had been pregnant as a young teenager and had a termination due to her youth, disinterest by the father, and lack of support. Abortion evokes controversy, guilt, fear, and intimidation both within society and within the hearts of women who find it necessary. Certainly, social mores and the associated emotions carry heavy influence both with the conscious and subconscious mind. Laura began to realize the significant guilt she still carried over many years. This caused feelings of unworthiness; she subconsciously felt that she did not deserve to get pregnant and was therefore punishing herself by not getting pregnant. Introspection led her to realize that the decision she had made as a teenager was the right one for her and did not make her a "bad" person. She also realized that she and her husband were deserving of a child. Thus, Laura was able to shed the guilt she had felt for so long and feel good about herself and her prospects for pregnancy. Sure enough, within a few months, Laura returned to confirm her pregnancy. Again, the healing took place within the inner self of the patient.

A third cause of nonphysical infertility is stress. Rita and Ben were typical of a couple who had tried everything in order to have a child of their own. Finally, after a couple of years, they decided to adopt a child. Five months later, Rita was pregnant. This is a common scenario. After adopting baby Susan, the pressure was off Rita and Jerome, and the couple was able to go with the flow of life and let nature take its course.

These examples illustrate how medicine, combined with open-mindedness and introspection, can help each couple achieve the best outcome for them, whether or not the result is a pregnancy.

Preparing for Pregnancy Holistically

Our society generally views pregnancy as a physical condition. However, I would venture that most people, especially those who have already experienced pregnancy and childbirth, believe that mind, body, and spirit work in concert during pregnancy as in any human endeavor. Therefore, it makes perfect sense to approach your pregnancy keeping all of these aspects in mind and giving each the attention needed in your particular case. Generally, the better shape you are in, physically, emotionally, and spiritually when you conceive, the easier and more fulfilling your pregnancy and delivery will be.

Medical Preparation

My advice to every woman is to find an OB/GYN she likes, one she can communicate with and relate to, before she gets pregnant. Make the effort to find a qualified, open-minded physician who is willing to listen to your desires, personalize the birth and prenatal experiences, encourage family involvement, and show genuine care and understanding for the unborn/newborn child and family. Unfortunately, these are sometimes hard to find, but worth it. A good relationship with your obstetrician will make it easier to work together toward the birth experience you want.

When you are ready to get pregnant, tell your OB/GYN, and have a thorough physical examination. Review your medical history and any medications you may be taking. In my practice, when everything has checked out and all seems normal, I tell the couple to simply stop using any means of birth control. Some obstetricians feel that a woman should be off of birth control pills for a few months before trying to conceive. I'm not convinced that is necessary. Some women get pregnant the first month after they stop taking birth control pills, others may take years.

No matter what conditions exist or how long a woman has been off whatever birth control she has used, when conditions are right for a pregnancy to occur, it will. When we simply let go and turn things over to Mother Nature, she usually does a good job of providing what we need, although that may not always be what we think we need or what we want.

Treasuring This Time with Your Partner

This should be a special time for a loving couple to become very close, physically, sexually, mentally, emotionally, and spiritually. Do what comes naturally, and enjoy the activity of conceiving life with your loving mate. Sex between two people deeply in love and wishing to conceive life is essentially a spiritual experience. Love creates love. What better start?!

Unless it proves necessary, I strongly advise against making love based on a watch or a calendar. Ovulation usually takes place midway between the start of two menstrual periods. A couple can keep this in mind without sacrificing any of the intended human experience of achieving conception. Keep as much love, fun, and joy as possible in getting pregnant!

Physical Conditioning

Obviously, you do not need to be an athlete in the peak of physical condition to have a baby. You also do not need to be thin. The average American woman is 5'4" and weighs 144 pounds. I have seen many overweight patients have good pregnancies. However, you can make your pregnancy and delivery much easier on yourself if you begin it in reasonable physical condition. If you have become sedentary, start exercising slowly and work up gradually. A daily walking program combined with some gentle stretching is a good choice for beginners. The point is to select an exercise regime that suits your lifestyle and physical condition and stick with it! Remember, a regular exercise program not only conditions your body, but it also helps your mental/emotional state for two reasons. You feel more confident in yourself when you are doing something positive, and the exercise helps clear your mind and relieve stress.

Walking and Stretching for Beginners

The most important part of beginning an exercise program is not how much you do but how regularly you do it. Walking is great cardiovascular exercise and easily achievable for most people.

Before you walk, make sure you have properly fitting athletic shoes, preferably designed for walking. Remember, if the shoes are not comfortable in the store, they will not be comfortable later on. Begin walking fifteen to twenty minutes daily and gradually work up to forty-five minutes to an hour. Try to walk in a pretty place where the air is clean. It will help your circulation, your muscles, and your attitude!

After walking is a good time to try some gentle stretching, because the walk will warm up your muscles. Just ten minutes of stretching a day will do wonders to improve your flexibility. Remember, never bounce when stretching; simply hold the position. Do what you can. If it hurts, do not do it. For an all-over stretch, try lying on the floor with your feet spread apart. Place your arms out to your sides and slowly raise them over your head. Hold this position for a minute or two, then put your arms down and repeat.

For a stretch you can do almost anywhere, anytime, stand straight against a wall. Extend your arms away from your body, parallel to the ground. Then slowly lift them over your head, hold for a minute or two, then repeat.

To stretch the lower portion of your back, try sitting in a chair and bending forward at the waist, so you are looking down at the floor. Hold your feet with your hands, and sit still for five minutes or so.

Nutrition

I cannot say enough about the importance of proper nutrition for both the mother and the unborn child. What you eat is the fuel for both of you. Unfortunately, our fast-paced, high-tech, fast-food society has changed many of our eating habits, to our nutritional detriment. So, developing good eating habits before pregnancy will be advantageous to you and your baby. Also, keep in mind that a combination of healthful eating and regular exercise will help you limit your weight gain during pregnancy. Let me emphasize, pregnancy is not the time to diet or lose weight. Also, going on a crash diet while you are trying to become pregnant is unwise. Try to modify your eating habits to include a more healthful balance of fresh, wholesome foods before you become pregnant and for the rest of your life.

Controlling Social Habits

Health-promoting lifestyle changes are best undertaken prior to conception so that pregnant mothers do not have to deal with additional stressful changes during early pregnancy. Social habits—smoking, alcohol, and drug consumption—can be detrimental to both you and your unborn child. All three can decrease your chances for conception, increase your chances of miscarriage, and heighten the risk for smaller than normal size babies, respiratory problems, fetal alcohol syndrome, an addicted baby, irritability, and other problems affecting the infant.

If you regularly use one or more of these substances at any level of consumption, chances are it will be difficult to stop. Additionally, the guilt you may feel for continuing these habits during pregnancy can have a significant effect on the you and your unborn child. Therefore, I suggest you break these habits before you get pregnant so that you can devote yourself to your pregnancy, instead of working on stopping addictive behavior or feeling guilty about it during pregnancy. There are many aids and programs available to help curtail cigarette, drug, and alcohol consumption.

Seeking Inner Peace

Pregnancy is a transforming experience and a rich opportunity for personal growth. A couple emotionally and spiritually prepares for pregnancy through introspection, seeking peace within themselves and harmony with each other, and thinking positive, loving, "pregnant" thoughts. Positive thoughts, meditation, and visualization techniques can help you get pregnant and can influence your pregnancy. So, think pregnant and visualize it.

Seeing and Believing

Visualization is a simple yet effective technique and a valuable part of the creative spirit we all possess. In short, it is a method of developing inner awareness, of realizing true feelings, of understanding the meaning of events in your life and of creating what you really want in your life. Does this mean that whatever you can dream up will come to pass? The difference between visualization and fantasy is that visualization involves a commitment to fulfilling true desires, whereas fantasy involves attaining unrealistic goals or good fortune without any effort.

Visualization techniques can be used in a variety of situations. Athletes, musicians, and actors often use visualization to help them achieve their optimum performance. Creating a mental picture of their most perfect performance helps them to focus on and achieve what they see.

Visualization can help to heal, to teach a skill, or to rehearse a coming event—all valuable aspects of the pregnancy and childbirth experience, from the initial desire to conceive a child to the actual delivery. The only prerequisite is a relaxed and positive frame of mind. Meditation can be helpful, but you can use any relaxation technique that works for you. If you do not know one, simply sit quietly, breathing deeply and slowly from your abdomen, concentrating on your breathing and allowing your random thoughts to pass by. When you feel quiet and relaxed but alert, create a vivid mental picture of yourself as pregnant. See the images clearly and in as much detail as possible. For example, picture yourself patting your abdomen, feeling the baby move, decorating the nursery, giving birth in a happy, loving environment, holding your newborn, and watching your family members' loving reactions. If your mind wanders, simply direct it back to your pictures. If negative feeling arise, experience them, and use them to help you figure out why a part of you resists moving toward your true desires.

Visualization can be particularly helpful in preparing for delivery. As biofeedback has measurably shown, the mind can have a powerful effect on the body. Dismiss the stories of long labor and excruciating pain that you have heard so often, and instead, work on visualizing your delivery as a joyful, cooperative effort between you and your child, with the assistance of your husband and/or family members, as well as your doctor. Remember, you must really want what you visualize. In order to realize it, you must recognize and act on the opportunities that come your way and put your will power and your energy into it, too.

For more in-depth information about visualization, see *Visualization, Directing the Movies of Your Mind*, by Adelaide Bry, or *Creative Visualization*, by Shakti Gawain.

After years of closely observing pregnant parents during the prenatal period, I have concluded that a newborn child's behavior, even in the delivery room, closely parallels the parents' personality traits and involvement in the pregnancy. A couple that is very involved in their pregnancy, that prepares for it and supports one another, as well as their unborn child, will usually have a calmer baby who cries little, if any, looks around the room, enjoys being held by its parents, and settles into the family very quickly. Prepared, loving parents project a "warm and fuzzy," calming and comforting atmosphere around the newborn. There is nothing mysterious about this. When adults are in a calm, loving atmosphere, we reflect it in our behavior, too. Conversely, insecure, uninvolved parents will often have fussy, dissatisfied babies.

To illustrate, I delivered a healthy baby to a couple having marital difficulties over the pregnancy. When their newborn son was given to the mother, the baby was calm and quiet. When given to the detached father, the baby grew fussy and irritable and cried, making the father feel even more uncomfortable and causing him to quickly hand the newborn back to his mother.

My long-term office nurse, who used to be a labor and delivery nurse, relates another connection. Pregnant parents who are nervous, lack confidence, and call the office with great frequency during pregnancy also tend to have the most irritable, colicky babies when they return for their postpartum visits. This makes perfect sense, since the way the mother or father holds the baby gives you insight into what you may expect of the newborn.

Thus, parents' prenatal involvement and attitudes are reflected in the conduct and outcome of their labor and delivery experience, as well as their newborn's behavior. Preparation, education, and positive attitudes are the keys to a happy outcome.

Conception is just the start of a pregnancy, and birth is just the start of many years of commitment to raising a productive, well-adjusted, self-confident, and unlimited loving person. Remember, "likes attract," so a strong, loving relationship that is created before conception is the best foundation to build your pregnancy on!

3

Communication

Use the Power of Love

A Positive, Loving Atmosphere

PREGNANCY is an ideal opportunity to explore the continuum of life. Many of the world's religions and cultural philosophies believe that life does not begin and end with birth and death. Many who believe that there is an eternal aspect of our individual selves—a soul, essence, spirit— also believe that even unborn babies are endowed with this spirit.

Years of research and close attention to details often overlooked in the birthing process have led me to realize the awareness, involvement, and responsiveness of the unborn and newborn. At a higher conscious level, they are no different from you and me. Unborns and newborns, though physically immature, possess individual spirits and freedom of choice, as we all do, and are influenced and affected positively or negatively by the thoughts and emotions that surround them.

Many factors can influence a birth outcome, starting at the time of conception and continuing through pregnancy to birth. While physical preparation and good obstetrical practices are essential, the most important factor in bringing a child into this world is love. Your loving thoughts and feelings actually create a positive atmosphere or environment around your pregnancy that can be actively used to achieve any positive outcome, even in a complicated situation. This does *not* mean that you ignore good medical advice. The two work together.

The power of love and prayer to help ailing patients recover has been gaining broad acceptance and understanding. I, myself, have seen many instances in which loving encouragement has coincided with a positive birth outcome. An early example came about ten years ago when I delivered a baby with an Apgar score of one at one minute, as well as at five minutes. This is a nightmare for any obstetrician and parent. It means that the baby showed almost no signs of life for at least five minutes. It was like a limp dishrag.

The initial emotion expressed or felt by all in attendance is fear. The obstetrician and nurses are the first to recognize the critical situation and must make a quick assessment and take immediate action. I stimulated the baby and gave it oxygen, a medication to counteract any possible narcotic effect. We pumped its little chest. We worked frantically to revive the lifeless infant. At such times, you barely have time to remember to pray and encourage the baby to respond and show signs of life. At times like this, your training takes over, while your subconscious works nonverbally with the infant's higher level of consciousness to evoke its needed cooperation.

The parents and family rallied around with loving, encouraging thoughts and prayers for the newborn. After what seemed like hours, but was actually only a few minutes, the baby started to show signs of life. From fear and deep concern came a glimmer of hope. Although the baby began to respond, I could not tell what the ultimate outcome would be. Often, these episodes do not turn out well. I recall a quick prayer of thanks for higher intervention and the baby's cooperation.

Amazingly, over the next day or so, this baby bounced back remarkably and went home in two days! I am convinced that the positive outcome was, in part, due to the loving, caring, and encouraging efforts of all involved. Love is the ultimate power, and your love for your child can have an awesome impact from the outset.

Bonding with your child does not begin at birth. It begins at conception, if not before. By developing, believing in, and using loving communication with your unborn child, you establish a bond and create a protective influence or "shield" with the unborn infant that can be the pivotal factor of a good birth outcome.

I often find prospective parents extremely receptive to the idea of communicating with their unborn child. Mothers, especially, intuitively understand that the child they are carrying is aware of them and responds to their emotions and surroundings. When I suggest prenatal communication to couples, most of the time the mother smiles, touches her abdomen, and says, "We already do that."

Occasionally, the mother will look over at her mate with an "I told you so" look. My suggestion can serve as encouragement or permission for the father to overcome his male hesitancy and open up communication. It is an interesting transition.

So, how can we communicate with the unborn child? It is easy; simply evoke and project loving feelings, support, encouragement, and reassurance. These feelings may be silent. They can but do not need to be verbalized. Unborn children cannot recognize individual language, but their essential selves understand the thoughts behind the words. There is power (truly) in the thoughts expressed in a loving and intelligent manner. For example, sitting quietly, think and feel: "We love you." "You are safe." "You are unlimited." "You are perfect." "All is well." Keep in mind that technique is unimportant. All you need is your heartfelt love and support.

Initial Reactions

When a pregnancy is confirmed, it is usually marked with a flood of emotions. Happily, most pregnancies are welcome, and couples can begin to establish a positive, loving atmosphere for their pregnancy. But, in some cases, unplanned pregnancies may be met with an initial negative reaction, or each partner may have a different reaction. Once the reality of the pregnancy settles in, couples may need to help one another overcome anxieties about the ensuing changes, the enormous responsibility, the financial burden, and all of the other "realities" of having a baby. My advice is to get your feelings out in the open. This is not the time to say what you think you are supposed to say, but the time to say what you truly feel.

Your true feelings, however, may not be your first reaction. Many people have a hard time getting in touch with their true feelings. Some find that quiet contemplation or meditation is helpful. Sometimes talking it out with someone you trust can help to clarify your emotions. One partner may need a great deal of patience and love to help the other. Supporting one another, dealing with negativity, and examining true feelings concerning the pregnancy helps couples to adjust to, accept, and become excited about the coming child. In order to illustrate, I will share two family situations with you.

Jim and Mary already had three children and had decided to have no more. Mary was taking birth control pills and was concerned because she had missed her menstrual period. When I informed her of the positive results of her pregnancy test, she nearly panicked, saying, "This was not supposed to happen while I was taking the pill! Jim is going to be really mad!" She left my office speechless, shaking her head in worry and disbelief.

Within a week, Mary returned with Jim. Both were in a state of denial mixed with anger and uncertainty over what to do. They reiterated that this "was not supposed to happen." They explained that

Jim's twenty-five-year-old brother was living with them, already causing family unrest due to his smoking habit and unruly friends. At their request, I discussed their options but advised them to make no hasty decisions. I urged them to go home and think about what they, not others, felt would be the best decision.

About a month later, the couple returned with one of their young children. They had given a lot of thought and prayer to their situation and had made several firm decisions. First, they had come to view the pregnancy as acceptable, even a blessing. Their children, too, were enthusiastic about the prospect of having a little brother or sister. Moreover, this pregnancy had given them the strength and fortitude to throw Jim's freeloading, inconsiderate adult brother out of their house in order to make room for the new arrival. Their enthusiasm grew with Mary's abdomen, and their mutual support was obvious. They eventually had a healthy baby. With four children, Mary decided to have a tubal ligation, to surgically obstruct her fallopian tubes in order to prevent future pregnancies, before she left the hospital.

Lori and Brian represent a couple with differing reactions. Lori and Brian had never really discussed in detail their desire to put off having children while Brian was in school. It was "understood." Lori was not too conscientious about taking her birth control pills and had already missed two periods by the time she came for a pregnancy test. On hearing the positive test results, her faced turned red, her jaw dropped, and she clutched her face in panic. When she regained her composure she said that she did not know what to do. Brian was working part-time and going to school. This was not part of their plan. He would be mad! She left feeling as though she were going to face the firing squad.

A few weeks later when Lori returned for her next visit, she was still showing signs of uncertainty and tension. She indicated that her husband did not take the news of the pregnancy well and blamed her for it. Although the initial explosion had passed, he was still upset, not speaking much, and sulking. I allowed her to vent her feelings and release some of her tension. Lori was actually happy about the pregnancy, or as happy as she could be considering the stress it had caused. She felt torn. Her relationship with Brian was good, but this pregnancy just was not in their plans. I suggested she give Brian some space and some time to reconsider the situation. Lori believed that if Brian would come around, they could adjust their priorities to accommodate the pregnancy and enjoy it. I urged her to send positive, loving thoughts to both her husband and her child, and I suggested she use her imagination to visualize the pregnancy proceeding as she would ideally like it to.

During the next few prenatal visits, Lori came by herself but indicated that they were now calmly discussing the pregnancy and the changes in their life that would probably need to be made. She was so excited the first time she heard their baby's heartbeat and wished Brian would share the experience. She cried a little out of her longing to share this incredible experience. I again cautioned her to let Brian come around at his own pace but to continue thinking positive, loving thoughts. A breakthrough came during the next visit. Brian took time off to come and hear the baby's heartbeat. I could tell he was still not totally committed, but he was there.

Over the following prenatal visits, Brian got more and more involved with the pregnancy and started showing signs of the doting husband and father-to-be. Lori confided that he had decided not to take any more night classes for the time being in order to devote more time to her and the baby. Fortunately, they received some financial assistance, which helped to take that burden off of them. Their childbirth instructor told me that both Lori and Brian were star students. And when the time came for labor and delivery, Brian came through with flying colors. They had a healthy baby and lovingly shared the experience.

Obviously, not all pregnancies, planned or not, have a happy, loving outcome. This is the reality of life and of human relationships. But, initial reactions can and often do change. However, even if the father remains uninvolved or abandons the mother, family and/or friends can rally around with supportive love and involvement, and the birth experience can still be positive, shared, and rewarding.

The Inside Story

As you think about and communicate with your growing child, follow his or her prenatal growth. Books such as *A Child Is Born*, by Swedish photographer Lennart Nilsson, allow us to see, via clear and detailed photographs, the progression of life before birth, from conception to delivery. Such pictures, combined with your intuitive sense and your imagination, can help you to visualize and empathize with your developing child and appreciate the interconnectedness of your bodies and your spirits.

For further reading on communicating with the unborn, I recommend *Communicating with the Spirit of Your Unborn Child*, by Dawson Church, and *Intelligence of Babies before Birth*, by David Chamberlain, Ph.D., both of which will give additional insight into working with your child before birth.

Prenatal Stimulation: Learning before Life?

Beyond loving communication with the prenatal child, many involved in the study of perinatal psychology believe that babies can benefit from special prenatal stimulation. The Association for Pre- & Perinatal Psychology and Health (APPPAH) has tracked studies done worldwide on the effects of prenatal stimulation. Such tests have revealed several benefits, including earlier speech and language development. One recent program to go under scientific scrutiny from the psychology faculty at the University of Valencia, provided 101 babies with taped violin sounds, arranged from simple to more complex forms, for up to ninety minutes per day beginning at about twenty-eight weeks of gestation. Mothers exposed their babies to the music for an average total of seventy hours. At six months of age, the babies in the experimental group were significantly advanced in their motor skills, linguistic development, sensory coordination, and cognitive development when compared with controls!

4

A Healthy Pregnancy

Nurture Yourself and Your Child

ONCE YOU KNOW you are pregnant, a million practical considerations start to race through your mind: choosing a caregiver and hospital, watching your health, altering your lifestyle, taking care of your growing baby, adjusting work schedules, preparing the nursery, dealing with sibling reaction, regulating finances, modifying insurance, etc. Sit down. Take a deep breath, and take things one at a time.

Choosing an Obstetrician

One of the first steps you will want to take is selecting an obstetrician and hospital. These two are very closely associated, but the primary emphasis should be placed on physician selection. There are several ways to go about selecting an obstetrician. Talk to your friends about their experiences. Find out what made their experiences special or unsatisfactory. You can ask your primary care physician and/or your gynecologist for a couple of referrals. A physician referral service can also give you information about several area doctors. If you are in a health maintenance organization (HMO) or if your medical insurance restricts your selection, try to interview several of the available obstetricians before making your choice.

Most obstetricians have privileges at more than one hospital, but it is usually wise to choose the hospital where the obstetrician does most of his or her deliveries. The physicians who actually practice at a given hospital are the primary determinants of the atmosphere, policies, and guidelines of the labor and delivery unit. A physician will individualize a patient's guidelines based on personal training, experience, and personality. Therefore, finding a physician who understands your desires and priorities is important.

Before you choose your obstetrician, think about the type of birth experience you would like. Read chapter 6 of this book to acquaint yourself with some gentle birth options. Visualize your delivery, and imagine the atmosphere you would like to feel around you. Then, sit down with your mate and talk it over. Make a checklist of the things that are important to you so you can discuss them when you interview the doctor.

The personality of the doctor is usually reflected by his or her office and staff. If you do not get a warm and concerned welcome from the staff, you probably will not get it from the doctor either. Be prepared with a checklist so you do not forget any of the questions you want answered.

Do not be afraid to ask all of your questions and do not accept anything less than complete, understandable answers. If you tolerate a doctor with a patronizing attitude, you may relinquish your control over labor and delivery choices. Think of your first visit as your chance to interview the physician and find out if you are compatible.

Interview with an Obstetrician

Here are some suggested questions for a visit to a new obstetrician.

- What is the obstetrician's general philosophy?

- Can family members come to office visits?

- Does the hospital have and use a birthing room?

- What is the atmosphere of the birthing room?

- Is there a whirlpool bath available during labor?

- Who is allowed in the room during labor and delivery?

- How much can the father, siblings, and family be involved?

- What techniques and alternatives are available for labor relief?

- How does the obstetrician conduct the actual birth?

- Can you take pictures or videos in the birthing room?

- What is done with the baby at birth?

- What happens if you need a cesarean delivery?

- In general, how does the obstetrician conduct a cesarean delivery?

- Can you have someone with you in the operating room?

- While you are in the hospital, can the baby stay in the room with you?

- How long will you be in the hospital?

- Who are your backup obstetricians?

A word of caution here so you do not have an unpleasant experience trying to interview a physician. Unfortunately, there are a fair number of obstetricians or physicians who will not feel comfortable being questioned about their philosophy and techniques. The "old school" taught that the physician is the total authority and not to be questioned. When initially calling a physician's office, make it clear that you want an interview. Be willing to pay for the doctor's professional time, as you may be charged for the visit. A great many doctors today are happy to be interviewed by prospective patients. So, if a physician's office staff is reluctant to schedule an "interview visit," move on to the next name on your list. Remember, you are not discussing the treatment of a serious disease. You are approaching a normal, natural healthy event that has been successfully repeated for thousands of years.

Most physicians follow the procedures they were trained to do, and change does not come easily. Before I began my metamorphosis, for example, I gave all laboring women an IV, enema, constant fetal monitoring, labor in bed, etc. I have individualized these procedures for many years now. Even though I was encouraging change, I will admit I was taken aback when a patient first came to me with a birth plan. I was not used to it, but it did not take me long to adjust. Now, I look forward to working with patients who take responsibility for, and put the effort into, a loving, gentle birth experience.

I will share with you probably the only request I have ever refused. It concerned the first underwater birth I did. The couple was very knowledgeable and knew what they wanted. They asked many questions and listed many requests, all of which we reviewed in detail over several office visits. Everything they asked for I already encouraged. At the end of the final early planning visit, the wife made a final request, "I would like my husband to do the actual delivery under water!" I hesitated for a second, contemplated the implications of her request, and calmly replied, "You just stepped over the line."

I reminded the couple that this was our/my first underwater birth and that we were already under the medical staff/hospital microscope, and they were waiting for something to go wrong in order to condemn this nontraditional approach.

I then turned my attention to the husband. With a sigh, he thanked me, saying, "I was afraid to try it anyway!" I pointed out to the couple that I would be practicing poor obstetrics if I were willing to let someone who had never had any training attempt a unique delivery, or even a traditional delivery.

So, while couples, at times, go to inappropriate extremes in trying to create a loving birth experience, it is perfectly appropriate to be firm about your reasonable requests. If the doctor is not willing to accommodate safe birth requests, be willing to go elsewhere.

Once you have found the "right" doctor for you—one who is highly competent, makes you feel comfortable, answers all your questions clearly, and treats you with intelligence and respect—you have begun an ongoing partnership with a valued medical health care advisor! The labor and delivery staff will usually follow this lead. Good labor and delivery nurses are usually "way ahead of the game" anyway.

Why Not Use a Midwife?

What about using a midwife instead of an obstetrician? Obviously, babies have been delivered far longer without physicians than with them, although a midwife or some other person usually assisted the laboring mother. A good midwife is certainly as capable of managing a normal delivery as an obstetrician. I have worked with nurses who were also midwives or nurse practitioners and found them to be knowledgeable, compassionate, and capable during labor and delivery. Even in physician-assisted births, the labor and delivery nurse and, of course, the mother do most of the work, while the doctor steps in near the time of delivery or when there is a complication.

Why would a woman choose a midwife over a physician? One reason often cited is that midwives tend to be more empathic, patient, and flexible in their techniques, particularly during labor and delivery. Some are willing to assist in home births. Midwives may also seem less threatening and intimidating to the patient. And, the cost for the services of a midwife, versus those of an obstetrician, can be considerably less.

The disadvantage of using a midwife instead of a physician is that they are not trained to handle some serious complications or perform cesarean surgical deliveries. While approximately 85 percent of pregnancies are uncomplicated and have a normal outcome, a midwife or an obstetrician cannot always know who may fall into the 15 percent who experience complications. Since some midwives do not have hospital privileges and cannot perform surgery, most responsible midwives seek out an obstetrician to whom they can refer complicated pregnancies. But, the midwife must be able to recognize when a pregnancy is not normal and immediately seek medical consultation.

There are two alternatives that can help solve this imbalance. The first that the physician try to assimilate the attributes that make the midwife more desirable. Years ago, I realized that a more flexible, caring, loving, gentle, family-centered approach leads to better birth experiences and happier outcomes for all involved. There is also no reason why a couple cannot have an individualized home-birth type of experience in the hospital, if they seek it out. This provides the best of both worlds!

The other alternative is to combine the efforts of the obstetrician with a well-trained, experienced midwife or nurse practitioner. This is beginning to become more common in medical institutions. While working in a small, rural Texas town, I teamed up with nurse practitioners in the local health clinic. The nurse practitioners took care of the uncomplicated prenatal care, and I took care of the deliveries and complicated pregnancies.

I do continue to maintain reservations about home deliveries, however. Emergencies can occur within minutes or seconds. Even in a hospital setting, it is sometimes a challenge to respond rapidly enough. All of those on the birthing team should be willing to make the effort to create a loving, gentle childbirth in the hospital. I have been a part of many, many such births and know it can be widely done.

Unfortunately, we cannot always tell which pregnancies will reveal unexpected complications or even life-threatening situations requiring immediate response. In my opinion, it is unfair to all involved to put the pregnancy at added risk.

Your Body Is Changing: The First Trimester

Pregnancy poses a significant physical challenge to a woman's body. Many physical and biological changes occur, affecting weight, body contour, hormones, blood volume, breasts, etc.

During the first trimester, some women experience what is commonly called "morning sickness." Please do not expect it to happen to you, because expectations can often be self-fulfilling. Nausea and vomiting may be a reaction to pregnancy hormones, or they may be due to a lack of vitamin B6 or glycogen (sugar). If nausea occurs, it is usually during the first three months of pregnancy and can come at any time of day. The traditional remedy, eating dry crackers or toast before getting out of bed, can be effective. Some women find that eating more frequent but smaller meals is also helpful. If all else fails, ask your obstetrician about prescription pills or suppositories. In extreme cases, hospitalization may be required.

Fatigue is a common effect of pregnancy changes. But excessive fatigue can also be caused by anemia, a fairly common occurrence during pregnancy. Ask your physician to check for anemia if you are concerned. During later pregnancy, you may tire more easily from carrying around your increasingly heavy load and blood volume! Rest and physical assistance is very important during pregnancy. The expectant father can show his compassion and love by sharing the load, especially if you have other small ones in your family.

As the baby develops during the first trimester, your expanding uterus presses against your bladder, causing the need to urinate more frequently. This occurs again later in pregnancy when the baby moves into the birthing position. This is common, so do not feel that anything is wrong, but if you have other urinary symptoms, such as burning or blood, consult your obstetrician.

Although you are under the care of an obstetrician or midwife, it is important to remember that you are your primary caregiver, in charge of your own diet, exercise program, stress management, and spiritual reinforcement—important aspects of your care during pregnancy are worth the time and energy you spend on them.

You (and Your Baby) Are What You Eat

A healthful diet is one of the most important factors under your control during pregnancy. In my experience, most mothers-to-be can describe a balanced diet as well as I can. So, in general, just follow common sense. Favor fresh vegetables and fruits, whole grains and lean proteins, such as skinless chicken or fish. During pregnancy, you will probably need more protein: six to eight ounces a day from meat, fish, poultry, eggs, beans, and dairy products. You will also want to increase your calcium intake. Try drinking several glasses of low-fat milk daily, or add low-fat dairy products, deep-green leafy vegetables, sardines, and salmon to your diet. Eat fewer fatty and fried foods, cut down on caffeine consumption, eliminate alcohol, as it can be damaging to the fetus, especially in early pregnancy, and drink plenty of water.

Do not completely eliminate the "fun foods" in your diet. Simply limit them so you will not create a craving for them.

While most of the vitamins you and your baby need can be derived from a healthful diet, your doctor will also recommend taking special prenatal vitamins containing folic acid, iron, and other important elements. Most prescription medications are safe to take during pregnancy, especially after the first trimester. If a medication is important for you take, it should cause no problem. Unless a drug is known to cause fetal problems and as long as it is important to your heath, it should case no problem, but check with your doctor. Make sure you also inform your obstetrician of any prescription medications you take. Do not take any other over-the-counter medications or additional vitamin supplements without first consulting your obstetrician.

During your pregnancy, keep track of your weight gain by getting on the scale once a week. About half a pound per week, or a total of about twenty-five to thirty pounds, is generally considered reasonable maximum weight gain. Keep in mind that your baby, the placenta, and the amniotic fluid only account for about seventeen to twenty pounds. That is how much weight you will lose when your baby is delivered. Of course, weight gain varies with the individual. My feeling is that while excessive weight gain is a risk factor during pregnancy, so is guilt. If you occasionally overeat, enjoy a good desert, or indulge in a fast food item, do not put yourself through a guilt trip. Use your common sense as guidance. Be kind to your body and your baby, but do not become a fanatic about it. Once you are home with your baby, if you maintain a healthful, balanced diet and take your baby for a daily walk, you should lose the extra pounds within a few months. The trick is to control weight gain during pregnancy so you do not end up stuck with extra pounds after each successive pregnancy.

Exercise Your Options

While starting out fit and healthy is a great advantage, the start of a pregnancy is not the time to undertake a major new physical training program. It is best to just continue a reasonable exercise regime started sometime before pregnancy. Physical conditioning can and should be continued through most, if not all, of your pregnancy. Generally, when pregnant, you should be able to do whatever exercise you did before. Although, as your pregnancy progresses, your level of activity may slow down as your body changes increase. Feeling fit and healthy will build your stamina and your confidence during labor and delivery, but use your common sense and do not overdo it. On the other hand, if you have become sedentary, try taking a daily walk. (See "Walking and Stretching for Beginners" in chapter 2.) Your level of activity is up to you. Listen to your body. It will let you know when you have overdone it. If it hurts, stop!

Women who are more serious athletes should consult their OB/GYN for guidelines concerning their particular sport. And, if there are any complications with your pregnancy, ask your doctor to suggest an appropriate program for you. In extreme cases, complete bed rest or hospitalization may be required.

Finding Your Bliss

Beyond traditional exercise, there are many methods of exercise, movement, relaxation, and stress reduction that can be helpful and effective for women at any time, but particularly during pregnancy when great demands are being placed both on the body and the spirit.

Yoga is an excellent discipline for keeping the body flexible and toned and keeping the mind calm. Certain yoga positions are especially beneficial during pregnancy and can be easily accomplished by most women (see "Stretch Like a Cat" on the next page). The practice of yoga postures emphasizes coordinating breathing with movement, while increasing strength and suppleness—great training for "natural" birthing techniques! Any woman who has studied yoga for some time before becoming pregnant will benefit greatly from it during labor and delivery.

Stretch Like a Cat

Certain exercises are specifically beneficial during pregnancy. One of the most common and easiest yoga postures to accomplish is called the "cat stretch." It releases lower back pain and helps maintain the back's strength and flexibility.

1. Get on the floor on all fours. Inhale, and arch your back, lowering the center of your spine and lifting your head up and back, like you are imitating a cat. Hold for ten seconds, then...

2. Exhale while you arch your back upward, rounding your spine. Pull your abdomen up and bring your head down between your arms. Hold for ten seconds.

Repeat the sequence once or twice.

Another aspect of the yoga discipline is meditation. While there are many types and methods of meditation, the basic concept is to quiet the constant action of your mind in order to understand your inner self. For some, prayer may be a form of meditation. For others, quiet contact with nature—watching the sunset, looking up at the stars, listening to the ocean's waves, staring at the embers of the camp fire—can achieve the quiet focus that is experienced in meditation. Others may find gentle music helps to calm and relax.

It may take more than a lifetime to reach true enlightenment through meditation, but it can be very beneficial to take time out from the constant roar that fills our heads. Concentrating on breathing and mentally repeating a sound or word helps to clear the mind and focus your thoughts on a single point. At first, your thoughts will wander, but, with practice, concentration will increase until the effort is no longer necessary for the single thought to remain (see "Thinking and Not Thinking" on the next page).

Yoga classes are given at yoga centers and, increasingly, at health clubs. You can usually take a sample class. Always inform the instructor that you are pregnant before taking a class, as certain postures should be moderated or eliminated during pregnancy.

Thinking and Not Thinking

It is said that meditation cannot be taught, it can only come by itself. However, here are some tips for getting started.

- Find a quiet place where you will not be disturbed.

- You may sit in the traditional "lotus" position on the floor with legs crossed, but it is not necessary. Sit comfortably in an upright chair if you like; but do not lie down, or you may fall asleep!

- Close your eyes. Start by breathing deeply into your abdomen for five minutes or so, focusing on the rhythm of your breath. Then, breathe naturally.

- After allowing your mind to wander for a few minutes, focus your thoughts on a sound or word you have chosen. Focus on this for as long as you can. When your mind strays, try to refocus.

- Be patient. It takes a lot of practice the keep thoughts focused. However, the time you spend will provide its own reward.

For more information on yoga and meditation, *The Sivananda Companion to Yoga,* by Lucy Lidell, has lots of illustrations and a special section on pregnancy. *The Complete Yoga Book,* by James Hewitt, covers every aspect and includes a chapter on the so called "effortless" Transcendental Meditation of Maharishi Mahesh Yogi.

You can also look for books or videotapes, and some cable or public television stations regularly air yoga programs. As with any exercise during pregnancy, do not do anything that hurts!

T'ai chi—an ancient Chinese discipline, sometimes called "meditation in motion"—works with the circulation to improve the flow of energy through the body. It also tones the body and puts the mind in a state of alert relaxation. The slow, fluid movements, done in a standing position, work with breathing, gravity, and balance. Once the technique or "form" is learned, the practice of t'ai chi can take as little as ten minutes twice daily and can be an excellent form of exercise for pregnant women due to its standing orientation, emphasis on proper spinal alignment, and capacity to relax and invigorate simultaneously. T'ai chi is difficult to learn from a book. Look around for a local class or videotape.

The modern term aromatherapy, meaning therapy based on the healing properties of the fragrance of plants, dates back to the 1920s. However, the use of essential oils goes back to ancient times. The essential oils used in aromatherapy are obtained by extracting oil from part of a plant: the roots, wood, leaves, flowers, or fruit. The aromatic, highly concentrated oils are believed by some to contain the essence of the plant's life force. Aromatherapists believe that essential oils can affect mood when inhaled, by triggering the release of relaxing or stimulating neurochemicals in the brain.

Essential oils can be used in a variety of ways: diluted in a "carrier" oil for massage; added to bath water; as an ingredient in skin creams and tonics; sprinkled on a tissue as an inhalant or in a bowl or warm water as an air purifier; or worn as perfume. The beauty industry is adding essential oils and other botanical ingredients in a wide array of products. While modern science has yet to fully explain the effects of essential oils, historical and anecdotal accounts are gradually being backed by scientific studies (see "The Essential Truth" on the next page).

I have not yet used aromatherapy in my practice, mainly because I have not found anyone locally who has expertise in the subject. But, I am convinced that there are benefits in a number of less traditional medical practices, such as aromatherapy and massage.

I am a big supporter of the use of massage therapy (MT). For those who are physically in tune with their body, it is a pleasurable experience and an effective stress reducer. I have used a massage therapist with my obstetrics patients, as well as infant massage for new parents. Massage therapy is used in several of my birth videos, and those who use it find it helpful for pain and stress relief.

The Essential Truth

Oils used for aromatherapy must be pure essential oils, not synthetic blends. High quality essential oils are increasingly available in health food stores or can be ordered by mail. Aura Cacia of Santa Rosa, CA, and Weleda Inc., of Spring Valley, NY, are reputable suppliers.

Essential oils must be diluted in a vegetable oil (not mineral oil) before they are applied to the skin. Sweet almond oil is frequently used in aromatherapy and can be readily found in health food stores. However, any vegetable oil without a heavy scent of its own (i.e., safflower oil or light olive oil) will do. Wheat germ oil is a good base if skin is very dry.

It is unwise to experiment with essential oils while pregnant, as some oils are contraindicated, but certain time-tested remedies are perfectly safe and may be helpful. Peppermint tea, for instance, can be effective in curbing "morning sickness" or heartburn. For those who become "smell-sensitive" during pregnancy, a few drops of rose, geranium, or lavender oil in a bowl of hot water will freshen and clarify the air. (Essential oils also have the added benefit of having antibacterial properties.)

Essential oils are frequently used in bathing. To lift the spirits, mix a few drops of lavender into warm bath water. To soothe the skin and relax the body, try mixing a few drops of chamomile oil into the bath. To cool and refresh, especially in summer, adding a few drops of peppermint oil to a tepid bath does the trick.

Essential oils can be used to condition skin and may help prevent stretch marks. Essential massage oils may also be used during pregnancy and labor. While aromatherapy "recipes" differ, these are simple, requiring few ingredients. You might try this one:

Massage Oil for Stretch Marks

- Twenty drops of lavender oil mixed in 2 fl. oz. (10 tsp.) of vegetable oil.

- Apply morning and night to abdomen and breasts beginning in the fourth month of pregnancy.

Massage Oil for Labor

- Ten drops of clary sage, five drops of rose, five drops of ylang-ylang mixed in 2 fl. oz. (10 tsp.) of sweet almond oil.

- A firm massage with the above combination of oils every so often during labor may help to relieve muscle pain and discomfort.

For more information on aromatherapy, here are three excellent resources: *The Art of Aromatherapy,* by Robert B. Tisserand, is widely considered the "bible" of aromatherapy for those interested in the history and many applications of this art. *Aromatherapy for Women,* by Maggie Tisserand, is written by Robert Tisserand's wife and contains practical, easy-to-follow information and applications specifically for women, including a chapter on pregnancy. *Aromatherapy for Common Ailments,* by Shirley Price, is beautifully illustrated with clear advice on everyday use and treatments.

Seek out the help of a well-trained therapist, preferably one who has had experience with pregnancy and birth, as there are certain techniques that are applicable to the pregnant patient. If you plan to use massage during labor, it would be helpful to start during your prenatal time. Fathers can certainly get involved and learn some basic techniques.

One unfortunate aspect of massage therapy is that insurance companies will usually not cover it. However, if you can afford it, I suggest you take advantage of it. And, as always, check with your obstetrician to make sure he or she has no specific objections.

Part II

Designing a Gentle Birth

5

Family Involvement

Engage the Help of Others

The Father's Role

THE FATHER'S ROLE during pregnancy and birth is often viewed as secondary to or as less important than the mother's role. And while on the surface this appears true, I would like to put strong emphasis on the benefits of the father's complete continued involvement from conception through birth and the rest of the parenting process.

There is no doubt in my mind that a father's active involvement in the pregnancy and birth experience is important to the comfort and well-being of both the mother and the newborn and helps to cement the bonds of the new family. I have known numerous fathers who have found their involvement during the pregnancy and participation in the miracle of birth to be a deeply moving experience, one without equal.

Every expectant father has the opportunity to be part of a team that ushers new life into the world, from conception to the vital first stages of child rearing and beyond. Those who fully take advantage of this chance are rewarded. However, there are fathers who, with a shrug of their shoulders, simply walk away from this unique opportunity. Such a man not only denies himself a wondrous experience, but, sadder still, he also deprives his wife, the new child, and the entire family of his involvement and support when it is needed most.

The role of the father should also be viewed from a higher plane in order to put its importance into perspective. The majority of our concerns during pregnancy and childbirth fall into the physical realm. This leads men to think that pregnancy is something that almost exclusively concerns the woman. Even the father's concerns usually surround the physical: the changes he sees to his wife's body; the baby's movements, sonogram image, and heartbeat; worries surrounding his reactions and his wife's pain during labor and delivery, etc.

This focus on the physical tends to exclude looking within and suppresses an understanding of our spiritual nature and the non-physical aspects of pregnancy and birth. This, in turn, prevents a true appreciation of the unborn.

Once open to the idea that there is an awareness and consciousness present in unborn babies long before birth takes place, fathers often see responses to their touch, to their voice, even to unspoken thoughts. I, myself, have witnessed changes in fetal movement, frequency, and location of fetal kicks and fetal heart rate in response to a parent's touch or voice.

Reluctant Participants

Often, the major question faced by the father-to-be is whether or not to be present at the birth. Many men feel reluctant because they dread the prospect of seeing their wives in pain during labor while feeling unable to be of help. The new father-to-be often wonders whether he can handle the birthing experience. He often feels self-conscious and ill at ease expressing his questions and concerns.

After many years in the birthing room, my response to such concerns is, "If you are not there, you are going to miss out on one of the most enriching experiences of your life." I tell them of the great joy a couple experiences together at the moment of birth and how seeing the father holding his newborn makes the birth an even more magical, more complete event for the mother. I also assure fathers-to-be that with all of the excitement and exhilaration, there is rarely a weak stomach or light head in the birthing room.

Fortunately, these days, the majority of men are taking a more active role during pregnancy and especially during the birth process. However, for too many, the involvement is moderate to minimal.

Unfortunately, our society historically has not encouraged male participation in childbirth or child rearing. Traditional male/female role separation kept many men from participating in the birth of their children. While this is changing, there are still many men who feel that once they have gotten their mate pregnant, they have proven their manhood and that is the end of their responsibility to the pregnancy…and to child rearing.

Economic pressures and expectations play a role, too. When a pregnancy occurs unexpectedly, at what seems to be an inopportune time, it often does not get enthusiastic support and causes additional stress to a relationship that may already be strained by long work hours and economic demands. This can leave each partner feeling isolated— the mother feeling unsupported and the father, uninvolved.

Employers also often do not realize or do not care about the long-term benefits of a father's involvement in the pregnancy, so they do not make it convenient or allow time for him to get involved. Our laws do not recognize the importance of a father's role and therefore do not influence employers to give men more family time, although most companies that have adopted family-friendly policies have benefited from them.

Even physicians sometimes do not understand the need for the father's active participation and do not encourage the future dad to come to prenatal visits or to get more involved. Regrettably, the father is not made to feel a vital, welcome member of the birthing team.

Encouraging the Reluctant Father

• Communicate openly about pregnancy and birth, and discuss all aspects, including any fears that might exist.

• Have other fathers who have taken an active role in the birth experience talk to the father-to-be and assure him that he will witness one of life's greatest miracles at the birth. After most fathers experience the birth, they usually say that they would not have missed it for anything.

• Do not force the father's involvement. Use gentle persuasion and patience in getting the father involved. Many fathers get involved at the last minute and are often the most enthusiastic participants.

• Schedule doctor appointments so that they are as convenient as possible for the father, taking his work schedule into account.

• If an ultrasound is suggested, schedule it at a time when the father is available. Being able to see your unborn child and his or her movements makes it feel real and binding.

• Create a good birth experience by working as a team. A wife should continuously reinforce her needs and the benefits of the husband's active role as a team member.

• Discuss expectations of the birth experience with the physician. Aim for the birth experience you want and do not be intimidated into retaining a doctor who does not want to work with the family.

• Select a hospital that understands and supports your desires and has designed its facilities and methods of operation with family convenience in mind.

• Think for yourself, and maintain a positive, loving attitude.

Getting "Dad" Involved

Getting the reluctant father involved should generally be approached slowly by both the wife and physician. An expectant mother's genuine enthusiasm can be infectious. And she can gently reassure her husband of the value of his support and the rewards for both of them.

The physician or midwife can also be especially influential in getting the father actively involved. If the father is ill at ease in an OB/GYN's office, seeking out a physician who will take the time and make the effort to work with the father and the family is an important early step for the mother. The decor and atmosphere of the office, coupled with the greeting from the staff and willingness of the physician to answer all questions clearly and thoroughly will provide important clues to the appropriateness of the "fit" between the doctor and the family.

The first major step is to encourage the expectant mother to bring her husband—and other family members—to prenatal visits. Hearing the baby's heartbeat is exciting for an expectant father and helps him feel involved. It also creates an excellent opportunity for the dad to have his questions answered by the physician. The father and siblings should feel welcome and comfortable. Look for an office designed with comfortable furnishings and a child's play area that can help to make the entire family feel at ease. Because I feel the doctor should stress the importance of the father's involvement, I make videotapes available to couples that address the importance of dad's active participation.

The obstetrician or midwife can also provide guidance and insights through furnishing handouts, books, and other educational materials.

A Team Approach

While in some ways society is moving in the direction of shared child rearing, many women today feel that they have simply gained more responsibility outside the home, while still maintaining responsibility for home and children. To realize real change, these issues must be addressed individually, by each couple, and by society as a whole.

There are numerous ways to bring the father into the birth and childbearing experience. First, both men and women should be encouraged to let go of stereotypical male/female role models. By embracing each other's preferences, accomplishments, and intelligences, rather than accepting traditional male/female roles, each couple can work out their own responsibilities. Men may be gentle, sensitive, and intuitive and may enjoy cooking and child care. Women may be rigid, physical, and logical and may enjoy a career and sports. If couples can make the most of each partner's strengths and abilities, they will be happier in their chosen roles and more likely to fulfill them enthusiastically. After all, the true inner self has no gender.

When children see this in their parents' lives, they will not allow themselves to be limited by imposed role models and inappropriate definitions. An acceptance of individual differences within shared responsibility helps to strengthen a couple's relationship and helps to create true partnership in bringing new life into the world.

I would like to note here that despite the demands of our fast-paced world, it is imperative that couples "stop and smell the roses" and reinforce their relationship. And, there must be continuous and effective communication. With a strong relationship, the couple is better able to take a proactive approach to their family and to plan a pregnancy and become jointly involved in childbearing and rearing. A planned pregnancy gives everyone—mother, father, baby, and siblings—an enthusiastic and positive start.

Remember, the true goal is not just to get the father into the birthing room. The goal is to get him voluntarily involved in the pregnancy, childbirth, and rearing. Preparation, education, and a positive attitude are the keys to achieving this goal. But, its realization will have a far-reaching effect on the family's relationship now and in the future and will have a small but profound impact on society as a whole.

Include Siblings, Too

Family involvement in the pregnancy and birth, of course, pertains to including other children in the family, as well as members of the extended family. Birth is a natural part of life; we were all born and many of us have become parents. It is our responsibility as parents to educate our children about human sexuality and reproduction. What better way to teach a child about pregnancy and birth than to offer your child an active part in the process of a loving, family-oriented pregnancy and birth. Sharing the experience in a wholesome, matter-of-fact way will help siblings feel good about the experience and provide them with a healthy, truthful appreciation for a loving pregnancy and birth.

How siblings respond to a pregnancy and the idea of a new person coming onto their "turf" varies greatly with each child's personality and age. It is important that parents lovingly help their children understand that the new sibling will not be a threat to their territory or to the amount of love and attention they will receive. A young child may not outwardly understand that there is no limit to the amount of love his or her parents can give. Gentle reassurance will help children believe that they will not lose any of their patents' love when the baby arrives.

Of course, parents, grandparents, friends, neighbors, and often, perfect strangers make a big fuss over the baby and shower the new arrival with presents. This is often perceived as a threat by an older sibling. One way parents can avoid planting the seeds of sibling rivalry or resentment is to encourage the child's involvement in the pregnancy and birth by including the child in activities surrounding the pregnancy. Make him or her feel like the important big brother or big sister whose efforts and support are needed, rewarded, and appreciated.

Parents can also remind friends and relatives that the older siblings still need their love and attention. Listen to your children, tune into their feelings, and observe their behavior. Children have many ways to convey their true feelings; you probably know them by now. If a child is ignored or neglected, resentment and negative attention-getting behavior will likely result.

Children are often smarter, more capable, insightful, and understanding than we adults realize. Children are also curious and inquisitive and tend to be more forthright and open when they express their feelings. I recommend that parents bring children—boys and girls—with them to prenatal office visits. I believe in providing an atmosphere that will make children feel free to ask questions, which should be answered simply, plainly, and truthfully. It is not uncommon for children to feel very protective of their mother and unborn sibling. They usually hold strong opinions regarding the baby's sex and, in my experience, are frequently correct! I always enjoy seeing their eyes light up when they hear their new brother or sister's heartbeat.

I recommend that parents sit down and watch my pregnancy and birthing videos with their children. The videos show actual births. The cesarean delivery shows a sibling happily interacting with the newborn. Watching the video prepares children for what happens during labor and delivery and provides an opportunity for children to ask questions. Do not try to force your child to be interested if he or she is not. Let them determine their own level of interest. If children—boys or girls—do express an interest in being present at the birth, I advise including them. If the child needs supervision, I request an adult, in addition to the father, be present. This adult can supervise the child so the father can give full attention to the laboring mother.

Many parents, friends, and relatives feel that children should not be involved in the delivery of a sibling. Many physicians and hospitals believe that children will "just get in the way" and discourage their inclusion. Some hospitals limit the number of family and friends or set an age limit for children. Some do not allow them at all, citing "hospital policy," as the reason. Certainly, there must be control over visitors, but I have found that these situations are self-limiting. Most mothers do not want a crowd in attendance; usually the father and perhaps one or two other people are present.

I have had experience with children of many ages being present and interacting at a sibling's birth. I have never experienced any problems as a result. The wonderful thing about young children is that they will be very honest with you and tell you exactly how they feel. They will also let you know how much they want to be involved. Unfortunately, some parents and grandparents do not think children can "handle" seeing a birth. Yet, in my experience, seeing blood at the birth does not bother most children; they watch what they want to see and turn their attention away from what they do not want to see. Children take in what their age and attention level permits, and they are refreshingly honest.

Each couple's insight into their own child's personality will help them decide what is best. I would like to encourage parents not to dismiss the thought of including their other children in the delivery. Children can handle more than many parents realize, and often they are intensely curious about birth. They also, unfortunately, are exposed to a lot of misinformation about birth through unrealistic, uncontrolled, melodramatic depictions on television and in movies. What better way to learn the truth about childbirth than to let them lovingly experience the birth of their sibling.

While family involvement differs with the ages and maturity of the children, the key to preparing siblings is to plan ahead so that they feel included instead of threatened; to be patient and loving when they act out their confusion; and to carefully listen to what they say. By involving your children in the birth experience, you give them the wonderful gift of a positive start on their own future, loving birth experience.

This reminds me of a couple, Troy and Mary, who had a five-year-old daughter, Sarah. As I do with all parents, I encouraged them to involve their daughter in the upcoming birth. When the time came for delivery of their second child, I was about to enter the birthing room when I saw their young daughter waiting outside, wanting to come into the room. As I was getting ready for the delivery, I repeatedly strongly suggested that they should let their daughter in to observe the delivery. They refused to let her see the actual birth but consented to let her in after the birth. I, of course, respected their decision.

During my rounds the next morning, the parents related that a short time after the birth their daughter reprimanded them for making her wait outside the birthing room door during the delivery! Wisdom from "the mouths of babes."

Young siblings often want to touch the newborn and get into bed with the mother and the baby. If there are no complications, I have no objection to this. Older siblings may be testing to see if they still have their share of access to and attention from their parents. Feeling included and receiving love so near to the new one's birth can be a strongly affirming and memorable moment for the child and the newly expanded family.

Older children can take a more active role during delivery. Some years back, I met June and Patrick. They had an twelve-year-old daughter, Marcia, and were soon to have their second, and last, child. Marcia was very involved with her mother's pregnancy. She came to all of the prenatal visits and attended Lamaze classes with her parents. When her mother went into labor, she came to the labor and delivery room with her and became "mother hen" for her own mother during labor.

When it came time for the delivery, I felt her dedication had really earned her the right to assist me. I asked her if she wanted to help me deliver her brother or sister. To say the least, she was very excited. I let Marcia put on a gown and the smallest pair of gloves we could find. (I do not wear a surgical hat or mask so that the baby can see full faces.)

I let her stand right next to me to "help" with the delivery and immediately hold the baby. We clamped the cord, and she cut it. She then handed her newborn sister to her mother. As she continued to be an integral part of the family dynamics in the birthing room, she was beaming from ear to ear with joy and pride!

Needless to say, this young lady made quite an impression on everyone present. I am sure when she eventually has her first child, she will likely have a very special birth experience of her own, due in part to her active and positive inclusion in the birth of her sister.

So, make your pregnancy and birth a family experience. Keep the father, siblings, and grandparents involved during your pregnancy and, if the excitement and enthusiasm is there, during the delivery, too!

6

Delivery Options

Find Out What You Want

Physical Growth and Change: The Second Trimester

DURING THE SECOND TRIMESTER, your body mirrors your baby's growth. As muscles grow and strengthen, the baby begins to lift its chin and flex its arms and legs. Tiny nails form, the bones produce blood, and the gallbladder produces bile. The external sex organs become more distinct.

The baby's facial features also start to develop. The eyelashes and brows appear, and teeth form under the gums. A downy hair, called lanugo, covers the face and body but will disappear before birth.

By about midpoint in pregnancy, a mother can feel her baby move within her. While the fetus has been moving for weeks, many women do not feel the movement distinctly until the baby's bones and muscles are harder and stronger. Now the baby's hair starts to grow, toenails form, and the nerve cells increase rapidly as the brain continues to develop. The baby may suck its thumb and can hear the steady beat of the mother's heart and the sounds of bloodflow and digestion.

Near the end of the fifth month, vernix caseosa, a fatty substance, forms to protect the baby's skin from the amniotic fluid. The fetus now looks like a tiny baby, about seven inches long, weighing ten to twelve ounces, and the baby's heartbeat can be heard through a stethoscope or doptone electronic listening device.

By the end of the second trimester, the baby is about nine inches long and weighs one and one half pounds. The baby's movement can be seen and felt!

During your pregnancy, you may or may not have a fetal ultrasound or sonogram. These procedures use sound waves and are a little like internal radar that shows an image of the baby on a small monitor. Gel is placed on the abdomen, and a scanning device is run over the abdominal wall. Numerous measurements are taken of the baby to help calculate the approximate gestational age of the fetus. Amniotic fluid volume and internal fetal organs are observed, and abnormalities are looked for. Ultrasound has proven very valuable and has allowed the medical community to gain insight into the unborn child and to diagnose ectopic (tubal) pregnancy and fetal abnormalities.

Ultrasound has been shown to be a safe procedure. However, numerous medical studies have indicated that it is not economically feasible to do an ultrasound on every pregnant woman if there is no medical reason for it. As with any other test given, there should be a medical justification for each ultrasound. Ultrasound tests can be done at any time during pregnancy, depending on the reason it was ordered. The most common reasons are: discrepancy between gestational dates and the size of the measured uterus; suspected multiple gestation; placental location; suspected slow growth rate; or fetal abnormality. Ultrasound is most accurate for determining gestational age between eighteen and twenty weeks.

Please understand if your doctor does not order an ultrasound. Be thankful; no ultrasound means that there is no indication of complication, and you are saving money as well! Some patients are willing to pay for an ultrasound simply to learn the sex of their unborn child. Many doctors have no objection to this, since ultrasound techniques are essentially harmless to both mother and child.

An ultrasound procedure is usually fun for the parents because they get to see the baby moving in the uterus and see the baby's heart beating. This brings a special closeness and reality to the pregnancy for the patient and other family members. The technician or radiologist will usually point out the baby's form. Some facilities will make a videotape or photograph of the ultrasound exam, thus providing a picture of the baby before birth! One word of warning, you will usually be instructed to drink thirty-two ounces of water without voiding before the test, so it can get a little uncomfortable; but it is well worth it!

Birthing Lore: Facts or Fiction?

As your silhouette indicates the dramatic changes occurring within you, your thoughts turn to the actual experience of birth. Giving birth is a milestone in a woman's life, one that connects her to the past as much as to the future. Every woman has heard the birthing lore of their family and friends; mostly heroic, horror tales of endless labor, incredible pain, and unexpected complications. It is easy to be influenced by the experiences you have grown up hearing.

For example, say your mother had a very difficult and complicated pregnancy and delivery, including considerable discomfort, and all during your childhood, she reminded you of the "horrible ordeal" she went through. Then, as soon as you became pregnant, your mother repeated the whole story in even greater detail, lamenting that her daughter would soon have to endure the "whole terrible experience." Naturally, you would not have a very positive attitude toward labor and delivery.

We often perpetuate the beliefs and experiences of those before us. Until the cycle is broken, the experience is repeated.

I have heard many variations on this theme from patients over the years. I can also offer a reverse example of a woman who told me she felt no pain during labor and delivery! It is not surprising since no one had ever told her she was supposed to experience pain!

You are not destined to repeat the experience of your mother, and at least to some extent, you can determine what kind of labor and delivery you will have. There are several factors within your control, and understanding and taking charge of those factors can help ensure that you, your family, and your baby will have the best, most comfortable (spiritually, emotionally, and physically) birth experience possible. But first, each couple needs to know what their options are and make decisions about what they want from their birth experiences.

How do you know what kind of birth experience you want? Labor and delivery is a process that you, your partner, and your baby go through together—an intense experience for all! Understanding exactly what happens to each of you during labor and delivery will help you understand what is important. In later chapters, I will go through the process with you. Childbirth education classes are also helpful preparation. They often teach and provide information on labor, breathing patterns, your partner's role, relaxation techniques, diet, exercise, cesarean-section preparation, breast-feeding, and the hospital labor and delivery area. You will, undoubtedly, also receive much well-intentioned advice from family, friends, and at times, perfect strangers. Before you start on the who, what, and where, first give yourself the opportunity to think about birth itself and time to quietly contemplate the experience of birth from the point of view of the mother…and the baby.

Childbirth: Two Viewpoints

In most cases, pregnancy is a normal, natural, healthy event and should be treated as such. Experience has convinced me that the more a laboring mother and her obstetrician work with Mother Nature, the better the outcome for both mother and baby. As I result, I have made many changes in my approach to labor and delivery.

When I first started in private practice, I could give impressive and medically logical reasons why the birth experience should be carried out clinically, the way I had been taught in medical school and residency. Such practices as using an IV, enemas, continuous fetal monitoring, and keeping fathers out of the delivery room (vaginal or cesarean), were easily justified, and I held to the taught philosophy and procedure.

After years of experience, I know that it is possible to have a loving, family-oriented, and individualized birth experience while still practicing good, safe obstetrics. It only takes a committed couple and a physician who is open-minded and supportive of the couple's wishes.

Birthing rooms with home-like settings have helped return the birth experience to the realm of "normal" and "healthy," rather than cold and clinical. Due to patient demand and the competitiveness of the health care field, many hospitals have modified their labor and delivery units to include birthing rooms and whirlpool baths, which can be very helpful during labor. Many hospitals have also adopted more liberal policies regarding family involvement. However, while these changes have helped to make birth a better experience for the laboring mother and family, there are other considerations that are more important to the newborn.

The most important preparation for the unborn child is your love. If the unborn child knows it is loved, then it knows all it needs to know. Those close to the pregnancy, including family, friends, and the medical team, should work to create a loving atmosphere around the pregnancy. Love is an energy and can be projected by voice, thought, or touch. So, simply touching the baby, via the mother's abdomen, is an effective way to get in touch with the unborn child.

We also know that during pregnancy, your baby's sensual awareness is continually increasing. She or he can hear many of the mother's internal noises, primarily her heartbeat. The baby is also aware of external sounds, such as the mother's voice and other sounds from the "outside" world, though they are all muffled through the surrounding placenta, amniotic fluid, and mother's body. In the later months, the baby can even perceive light if the mother's abdomen is exposed on a bright day. An unborn baby lives in a liquid, temperature-controlled environment with a protective layer covering the skin, even still touch is another way it perceives its world.

Obviously for the baby, leaving the dark, warm, quiet, liquid environment of the uterus by a process of frequent squeezing sensations (contractions), and then moving through a rather tight, narrow tunnel (birth canal) out into a very different environment (often bright, loud, and cold) has to be quite a bombardment of new, unfamiliar stimuli to say the least! Yet, during a typical hospital birth, a newborn is subjected to bright lights, jolted by loud voices and noises, chilled by a foreign environment, and roughly stimulated and handled! Also, the newborn is then whisked off to a strange, brightly lit room (newborn nursery) for confinement with perfect strangers for up to its first four hours of life. Is this the kind of birth experience you had in mind? I feel strongly that every effort should be made to create a gentle physical and emotional experience for the baby to remember and be influenced by.

In his controversial 1975 book, *Birth without Violence,* Frederick Leboyer focused awareness on the baby's painful physical experience during birth and just after. He also outlined how, with relatively simple adjustments, babies can enter the world more gently, avoiding such "birth trauma." Leboyer advocated such practices as low-level lighting to help the newborn adjust to this new, light-filled world; quiet, so that the newborn is not startled by the louder, sharper sounds of the new environment; placing the baby on the mother's abdomen immediately upon birth for warmth and to help ease the transition from mother to outer world; leaving the umbilical cord uncut until the transition to lung breathing is made; and placing the baby in a warm-water bath to allow relaxation.

This approach to birth was highly controversial only a couple of decades ago! Yet, while we continue to understand more about the world of the unborn child, gentle birthing techniques are still not widely practiced today. It is my hope to spread the word that a gentle, loving, essentially non-traumatic birth is important, available, and can be done within the guidelines of good obstetrical practice.

Most pregnancies, approximately 80 to 85 percent, are uncomplicated and leave room for flexibility in the birth experience. Below are some safe, innovative birthing options that should be implemented whenever possible.

Allow Family Members to Participate

For many years, I have realized the importance of support for the laboring mother and the unborn child. I have encouraged the father's, family's, and friends' active participation and support. Years ago, and in other cultures, pregnancy and birth was a tribal, community, or family affair.

In my own practice, I leave it up to the couple to decide who will be present in the birth room. The number of guests has ranged from one to about fifteen! The usual number is two or three. I have never had a problem with those present and would not allow an interruption to the birth experience. As a doctor, if your attitude is that guests will not be a problem, they usually are not. I try my best to let childbirth be the couple's experience. My role is just to make sure everything goes smoothly, medically. However, hospital policy on children's presence in the labor room varies. Many hospitals try to limit the number of people in the room to about two visitors. Obviously, the size of the birthing room plays a part in the decision.

Most general policy for protocol in labor and delivery is determined by an obstetrical committee composed of the physicians who deliver babies at the given hospital. The specific protocols are somewhat individualized by each physician. I personally wrote specific protocols for the conduct of labor for my patients' use of the whirlpool bath during labor and underwater births. It is rather rare that an individual physician will write a specific protocol for his patients, but change and improvement need to be defined. Some of my individual protocols, such as the two mentioned above, had to be approved by the obstetrical committee.

Combine a Home-Like Setting with Medical Technology

A warm, home-like setting helps to create a family atmosphere. Some years ago when the labor and delivery rooms of the hospital at which I was practicing were remodeled, a female obstetrician and I made time to select the colors, furnishing, and decor to assure a home-like "feel." But the birthing room's real advantage is that it also provides the medical facilities that might be required in case an emergency situation occurred without warning, which is not a rare event.

This point sums up an important concept. Create an atmosphere in which you have the best of two worlds: the loving, family-inclusive setting of a home delivery and the immediately available technical support of modern obstetrical principles in case of a rapid onset of a life or death emergency. Every obstetrician knows well how rapidly this type of emergency can occur, and he or she wants to be able to appropriately respond with everything and everyone readily available.

Use IVs, Enemas, and Fetal Monitoring Only as Necessary

The way I was taught in medical school, admission procedure included an enema, IV insertion, shaving around the vagina, no oral fluid or food intake, and staying in bed with continuous electronic fetal monitoring (EFM). It all seemed necessary until I was willing to try it without some of these "necessities." Now, I believe the way to approach these points is to individualize their application. I can now say, with many years of hindsight, that this individualization has in no way compromised my birth outcomes but has only added to a more positive atmosphere and outcome.

Assist but Do Not Restrict the Laboring Mother

Most everyone would agree that labor is hard work. Everyone responds to it in their own way. Therefore, removing unnecessary restrictions on the laboring family allows individual preferences to maximize the mother's comfort. In uncomplicated labors, mothers can get up, walk around, and/or use the whirlpool tub, if available, as they choose. Another useful technique is using a Transcutaneous Electrical Nerve Stimulation (TENS) unit, which uses electrodes attached to the mother to help block nerve stimulation to the uterus and cervix, thereby minimizing labor discomfort.

Create a Tranquil Atmosphere during Birth

This benefits everyone present, the newborn especially. Parents may choose to play soothing music. All present should keep speech tones soft.

Eliminate Bright Lights during Birth

Low-level lighting is easier on the emerging baby and does not interfere with a medically safe delivery. I have never understood why a laboring mother should have to lie on her back and stare directly into a bright ceiling light over her bed. I am usually somewhat offended when I walk into a brightly-lit labor and delivery room.

Allow Time for the Newborn to Be with the Family after Birth

We know the importance of physical bonding between mother and child. For a new mother, father, and infant, this is a magical moment and should not be rushed, unless complications occur. Believe it or not, most newborns are very safe with their parents in the labor and delivery room. The newborn is exactly where it came here to be— with its parents.

Create a Loving, Caring Atmosphere in the Birthing Room

The medical team, as well as the family, needs to recognize the intensity of the experience for the newborn and respect his or her right to a gentle, loving entry into this world. In my birth protocol, I ask all those involved with the birth to leave any problems and negative thoughts outside the labor and delivery room. This certainly applies to friends and family members. Occasionally, there is family friction that develops and this has to be eliminated.

Include Gentle Birthing Elements in Cesarean Deliveries

Even in a cesarean delivery, it is possible to include the father and adapt the operating room atmosphere for the newborn by dimming or turning off the ceiling lights, speaking softly, and playing soothing music. In cesarean-sections, just before delivering the head, I usually rotate the surgery site lights a little to avoid blinding the newborn. In uncomplicated cesarean deliveries, mother and baby can still be given time to bond, and husbands can offer loving support during the surgery and help with the baby after birth.

Getting (at Least Some of) What You Want

How can you assure a more family-oriented and gentle birth experience? It starts by taking responsibility for your child's birth. This means first making a commitment to pursuing what you want, then finding the right practitioner—one who understands and shares your feelings and desires and who can clearly explain your options.

As a society, we are used to deferring to medical practitioners. However, seeking out a doctor who is willing to listen to your desires, personalize the birth and prenatal experiences, encourage family involvement, and show genuine care, love, and understanding for the child and family is worth the effort.

This may not be easy. You may not find a physician who meets all of your criteria, but your persistence will at least assure you that you have made the best choice for your family. This is part of committing yourself to the effort that will ensure the best possible outcome.

When you approach the physician, be reasonable in your requests. Work with the obstetrician, but do not give up on a gentle birth plan. Be willing to speak up for what you want, and do not make compromises that you are not comfortable with. Remember, it is your birth experience.

If the physician you have chosen turns out to be rigid in his ideas and is offended by your suggestions, you have obviously selected the wrong obstetrician. Do not be afraid to change. Staying with an obstetrician who does not respect your desires will become a bigger problem...or a regret. Understand that you, the patient, will greatly help create the necessary changes in attitudes and approaches to birthing so that a gentle, loving birth experience becomes standard practice. When enough patients walk out of an obstetrician's office because the physician is not willing to change, then the practice of obstetrics will slowly start adapting to the patient's desires. Do not underestimate the power you have to help encourage change. If you do not make the effort, you have no right to complain.

In my own practice, I have noticed that more women are willing to speak up for what they want. I enjoy it when a patient comes in with her list of requests. In fact, it was through the request of a couple that I undertook my first underwater birth.

Unfortunately, I must also point out that many patients do not speak up about their own birth plans since they have given no thought to one. Many patients have not given any thought to getting pregnant, much less to a birth plan! This is partly because most couples do not realize that they have any choices regarding labor and delivery. I am confident that this will change as the public learns more and becomes more aware of their options.

It took me a few years to realize and accept the fact that as a doctor I can offer couples information, but I cannot make them act on it. As I tell my patients, "I can help you have a very good birth experience, but I cannot prevent you from having a bad one." As a doctor, I assist and encourage each couple's effort and do my part to add loving encouragement when and wherever I can.

Among expectant couples, the level of interest, involvement, and desire for insight varies widely, from detachment to full commitment. Of course, I always enjoy working with couples who are excited, open-minded, eager to learn, and interested in doing all they can for their unborn child. Such couples are usually rewarded by the creative effort they put into their pregnancy and birth experience.

Remember that visualization can help you imagine and prepare for the delivery you want. Just as an athlete visualizes performing an event perfectly, the expectant mother can rehearse childbirth as she would like it through visualization. The clearer, more detailed, more positive picture you can evoke, the better. Find a quiet space. Steer your mind away from fearful thoughts. Work with your baby; assure your child that all will be well. Picture yourself and your baby feeling ready and working together for a smooth delivery. Picture your baby entering the world gently to a loving reception. Picture yourself holding your healthy baby, rewarded by the effort it has taken you both.

I will always remember one example of creative childbirth, because it was a case of a patient overriding my obstetrical thinking and shows the power of desire and visualization. Thank goodness it had a happy ending.

I had a patient who I diagnosed with a bicornate uterus (a heart-shaped uterus with a wall part way down the middle of it). This resulted in difficulty getting pregnant. I did major surgery on the uterus to remove the wall, which required the entire uterus to be surgically opened, thus leaving a large scar and possible weakness in the wall of the uterus. I was very happy for her when she got pregnant a number of months later.

Due to the significant surgical scar in her uterus, I informed her, as any obstetrician would, that we needed to plan for a cesarean delivery to avoid the risk of uterine rupture, which could be a life-threatening complication. We seemed to have a good understanding.

At term, she came into labor and delivery having contractions. As usual, I did a pelvic exam to check for cervical dilation. To my shock, I found her to be almost completely dilated (near ten centimeters)! I had said I did not want her to risk labor, but I immediately sat down to discuss the situation in detail with her and her husband. I told them that despite my earlier warnings, she had almost completed labor with no complications. If they wanted to proceed with an attempted vaginal delivery, I would work with them closely. We soon achieved an uncomplicated vaginal delivery, and I was relieved! I was happy to observe this safely achieved alternative, but I hold to my original philosophy of an elective cesarean in such cases. Because the specific circumstances of this case were uniquely favorable and the parents fully aware of the risks, I cooperated with the parents' desire to complete the vaginal birth.

After the delivery, I spoke with the patient about the experience and was given insight into the power of visualization and wishful thinking. She confided that she had always seen herself having a vaginal delivery and had thought a lot about it. When I asked how long she had been thinking about it, she answered, "Most of my pregnancy." I suggest you put your power of visualization and determination to safer pursuits.

Another brief example of determination centers on anticipating the use of forceps. It is common for a laboring mother who has seemingly "stalled out" to deliver soon after forceps are brought out, unwrapped, and "rattled" a little. Her determination to deliver without forceps gives her body the "jump start" she needs. So do not underestimate the power of visualization and determination. Use it to your advantage.

My message to every expectant couple is that it is up to you to create your own birth experience. Contemplate birth, learn about options, discuss it in detail with your spouse, find a sympathetic physician, keep communicating with your baby, and visualize your ultimate birth experience.

7

Delivery Planning

Make Final Preparations

The Inside Story: The Third Trimester

BY THE THIRD TRIMESTER, your body reflects your rapidly growing child. As the baby's body grows more in proportion with the head, moves and shifts look and feel more pronounced. The unborn child grows increasingly cramped within the tight quarters of the uterus. The baby's senses are starting to function. Hearing becomes more acute. Eyelids slowly open and are soon able to detect changes in light and shadow. Taste buds develop. Hands start to grasp. As fat increases, the baby's wrinkled skin smooths out. The lanugo and the vernix caseosa are almost gone.

Within the last trimester, the mother begins to pass protective antibodies into the baby's bloodstream. This immunity lasts a few months after birth and is fortified by additional antibodies transmitted during breast-feeding.

As delivery nears, the baby continues to move and stretch. Near the end of the ninth month, the baby may turn, head down, facing the mother's back, in preparation for delivery.

Preparation's Payoff

Since childbirth is a natural process that women have been going through for thousands of years, you may have wondered, from time to time during your pregnancy, why you should go through so much planning and preparation. Why not just let it happen? The answer depends on the kind of birth experience you want. Like most things in life, you will get out of the experience what you put into it. But let's look at some of the most obvious benefits of preparing yourself for the event.

Any physical conditioning you choose, along with the mental discipline and focus that accompanies it, will pay off by giving you better control over your labor. Visualization will help you to expect a good experience. Working ahead of time with your support team, usually lead by "dad," will help build each team member's self-confidence as well as team confidence. Reassuring and preparing the unborn child with your encouragement and love will continue to reinforce the bond you have established. Having a comfortable rapport and good communication with your obstetrician will reinforce your confidence in him or her and will help you to understand and feel comfortable with the process of birth, eliminating fears of the unknown.

By now, you should have a good idea of your obstetrician's philosophy and protocols. You and your obstetrician should have established a clear understanding regarding family involvement, the birthing room atmosphere, the actual birth procedure, and how the baby will be handled. You have chosen a hospital and are probably taking childbirth classes.

I strongly suggest childbirth classes, even for repeat parents if it has been two or more years since they last took one. Many classes include a tour of the labor and delivery (L&D) area of the hospital. This tour is especially informative for new parents or those who are new to the hospital. Many hospitals now have LDR rooms, which stands for labor, delivery, and recovery. This means a patient can stay in the same room through all three stages of her birth experience. Many LDR rooms are furnished to look like bedrooms and provide the benefits of a home-like atmosphere with the safety features of an emergency facility readily available for the occasional times they are needed. Visiting will familiarize you with the area so that it will not be a strange unseen place when you come into the hospital. While touring the area, note whether there is a waiting room for children and family members, and ask about visiting policies.

Getting Down to Specifics

If you have not already done so, now is the time to build onto your earlier preparation and think about some of the specifics of the labor and delivery experience. Here are suggested questions for you to consider and discuss with your obstetrician.

- What should you bring to the hospital?

- Should you go directly to the labor and delivery area?

- What happens upon admission?

- Do you have to stay in bed with continuous electronic fetal monitoring?

- Do you have to have an enema and an IV?

• Do you have to be shaved? If so, can a "mini-shave" be used?

• Does the hospital have a birthing room?

• Does the birthing room have a whirlpool bath?

• What techniques and alternatives are available for labor relief?

• Will you be made aware of any potential or existing concerns or complications?

• Can the father (or someone else) be with you during labor and delivery?

• What happens if you need a cesarean delivery?

• In general, how does your obstetrician conduct a cesarean delivery? Can you retain a "gentle birth" atmosphere?

• Should you talk to an anesthesiologist (if you think you may need their services) before you go into labor?

• What are the obstetrician's feelings about episiotomy?

• How long will you be in the hospital?

• Which pediatrician does your obstetrician recommend?

Your obstetrician should be willing and able to answer these or whatever questions you may have. Unfortunately, some physicians still do not feel they can make time to answer a lot of patient questions. Personally, I feel that educating the patient and answering their appropriate questions is one of the physician's most important responsibilities. You would not buy a car from a salesman who would not answer your questions, so why settle for less when it concerns an event of far greater importance in your life? Patient demand is what brings about change. Do not be intimidated by your physician, she or he is there to serve you.

Pain Perception, Pain Management

An important aspect of childbirth that should be discussed ahead of time with your obstetrician is how to handle labor contractions. I am purposefully doing my best to avoid the word "pain" because I do not want to plant the idea in your mind that you will have pain. Each woman's response to a potentially painful stimulus, such as a firm labor contraction, can be, and is, quite varied. From person to person and culture to culture, there are dramatic differences in response to essentially the same experience. The factors that play a part in determining one's response to pain (other than the severity of the causative stimuli) are human anticipation, attitudes, and cultural traits.

Some people handle a painful stimulus in a controlled manner, while others may be completely out of control with the same experience. In Brigette Jordan's investigation of childbirth in the Yucatan, Holland, Sweden, and the United States in her book *Birth in Four Cultures*, she compares both the perception and the management of pain in each of these different cultures.

Jordan notes that the experience of pain is, at least observationally, more apparent in American obstetric wards than in Sweden, Holland, or the Yucatan. This, she believes, stems in part from the fact that in

American hospitals the decision to administer pain medication is made by the physician. Thus, the laboring mother must convince the obstetrician of her need for pain relief, leading, Jordan notes, to a comparatively high level of vocal and physical expression of pain in American obstetric wards.

In Sweden, by contrast, where decisions regarding pain relief are largely up to the mother, and pain medication is used fairly routinely, Jordan noted a quieter atmosphere of intense concentration, rather than vocal panic.

You need only watch animals to see the birth experience completely in concert with Mother Nature. You see a quiet, controlled determination of the experience, working with, not against, nature's time-proven and ever-evolving techniques. It seems that the "more evolved" human, who has moved away from nature, focuses on the pain aspect of the experience instead of the birth. Watching a laboring animal, there is no doubt that she is working very hard, but you can also see that she is well in control.

Interestingly, in Jordan's study, both Dutch and Yucatan women, while very different culturally, tended to view birth as a natural process that should be interfered with as little as possible. These women expected and accepted the pain that can accompany childbirth but viewed it as a normal and passing aspect of the process, not its focal point.

So, if you have been influenced to expect a certain experience, positive or negative, you will probably have that experience. In my practice, I have seen a great variety of responses to labor contractions. Typically, women who are the least prepared mentally, physically, and emotionally have the worst experiences. Those who fight labor, who do not work with nature, and who are not prepared for labor have the greatest difficulty controlling the process and therefore amplify the discomfort.

However, this is not to say that you should not use anything to help keep you more comfortable during labor and delivery. You should be aware of the alternatives available and select what best meets your needs. This is your birth experience and you have choices. Do not concern yourself with outside advice and opinions; choose what is good for you by discussing it with your obstetrician.

Among the agents and techniques available to help you with contractions, two will affect the unborn child: general anesthesia and injectable pain medication. I do not use general anesthesia during vaginal deliveries. In fact, I have only used it in emergency cesarean delivery situations. I also do not strongly advocate injectable pain medication, because I do not like to sedate unborn babies, although, overall, it usually causes no problems with the baby. Because I believe that a woman should have choices (within medically safe limits, of course) and some patients do request injectable medication, I will comply. However, I do not believe it is appropriate to give medication unless it is specifically requested, and I do restrict injectable medication near the time of delivery since you tend to get sleepy babies, due to the fact that the pain medication does not have time to metabolize or break down quickly enough.

Happily, there are other alternatives that have little if any direct effect on the baby. Some are widely available, others are slowly gaining acceptance, and still others have not yet gained recognition from the American obstetrical community.

Epidural anesthesia is a spinal type of anesthesia that is usually injected through a tiny plastic tube into the space around the sac (dura mater) that surrounds the spinal cord. Epidurals are usually given when the cervix is dilated to about five centimeters and the woman is making good progress with her labor. Some physicians claim it may slow labor a bit, but I am not convinced that there is a significant delay with epidural usage. It does provide excellent relief from the discomfort of labor contractions, while still allowing the patient to push after she is completely dilated. Epidural anesthesia is the appropriate choice for some patients delivering vaginally, and is the method of choice for cesarean delivery.

Natural, noninvasive, yet extremely helpful, techniques include the use of the warm whirlpool bath and massage. Many women fight against the process of labor, intensifying their discomfort. A warm whirlpool tub and massage techniques can allow the woman to relax somewhat and work with the natural forces of labor. Patients who have chosen these techniques usually find them very helpful. I have used these in a number of my deliveries.

The TENS unit is a nerve stimulator that helps block the nerve impulses that cause pain. This small, battery-powered unit is about the size of a beeper and has one or more wires connected to it that lead to a small skin electrode patch. By sending electrical impulses to a certain nerve area of the body, it blocks a major portion of the pain sensations. In the United States, it is mainly used by physical therapists for reducing chronic pain. The patient can control the strength of the impulse, and it is safe for use during labor. When a TENS unit is used, the physical therapist comes to the labor and delivery area, applies the electrodes, and instructs the patient on its use. Several of my patients have found it to be quite helpful in reducing the pain of contractions.

When I first began using the TENS unit, some concern was expressed about electrical hazards. However, the power is so minimal, about equal to a nine volt battery, that it is not a realistic concern. Most American obstetricians do not use TENS units, preferring to stick with the traditional means of pain management, which tend to be more invasive. However, the TENS unit has been widely used in Europe for help during labor and has been found to be about 70–85 percent effective.

Two other alternative means of pain control that have, or could have, application to the laboring patient are hypnosis and acupuncture. Both have been used in Europe and China, either for vaginal delivery or for surgical procedures. Unfortunately, these techniques have been used very little in the United States. I hope they will be objectively evaluated for labor use, as they are noninvasive and hold promise for laboring mothers.

Acupuncture, which is based on the body's invisible energy grid, involves inserting very fine needles at appropriate points to interrupt pain sensations. I have not yet had the opportunity to witness the use of acupuncture. However, I have read of major surgeries in China that used only acupuncture for anesthesia. Apparently, the use of acupuncture also reduces the surgery recovery period as well as reducing the frequent intestinal side effects. Acupuncture specialists have assured me that it could be quite useful during labor.

We have all heard of the theatrical and therapeutic uses of hypnosis. Its usefulness reveals yet another aspect of the power of the human mind over the body. Hypnosis is simply a more direct access to the subconscious mind. Under hypnosis, the mind can block pain sensations. I have read about cases of women who underwent cesarean sections using only hypnosis! Of course, with hypnosis, there are none of the side effects of drug anesthesia.

Talk with your obstetrician about dealing with contractions before you are in labor. If you are interested in the possibility of using an "alternative" method of pain management, and live in an area where a specialist is available, talk to your obstetrician about it. In truth, there are always obstacles to using a new procedure in the labor room, and most obstetricians will not try. But there are those who will. Find out your options. It is part of preparing yourself for labor and will help you to feel in control, build your self-confidence, and dispel your fears of the unknown. Avoid dwelling on the negative. Work with what is possible, and use your imagination positively to reinforce the birth you want and to encourage and reassure your unborn child. In time, and with patients' insistence, many such "alternative" techniques will be evaluated and used during labor.

Listening with Your Heart

During the last trimester, the unborn child is obviously physically developing, but it is also gaining insight and familiarity with those close to the pregnancy. Your spoken and unspoken thoughts, directed to your unborn child, are your true connection. Do not hesitate to explain what is happening to your child in an intelligent and loving manner. Your continued, loving communication and reassurance is helpful preparation for the baby and for you.

You can also learn things from your unborn baby by listening, not with your ears but with your heart, in a quiet, introspective, and interactive way. Go within yourself, and focus on the baby and your love for him or her. We have all heard of "mother's intuition." Just carry it one step further. We are taught to rely on our physical senses, but we also have the potential to develop our intuition. Have faith in your inner self, trust it, and work at developing this "sixth sense." Do not expect booming voices from within. Be aware of quiet, fleeting insights that you might normally dismiss. If you give yourself a chance, you may be surprised by the amount you can sense about your child.

While you are thinking about the baby, I would like to make a few comments about preparing the baby's room. This is an enjoyable and loving project for most couples, particularly for a first child. Safety is the primary consideration. Keep in mind that the baby will grow quickly, and set the room up so that your child will be safe when he or she begins to move around. Ideally, the room should also provide a fair amount of sunlight and pleasant colors. Do not feel restricted to pastels; use your creativity! Also, do not feel you have to fill your baby's room with toys and equipment. Babies receive ample stimulation from a fairly simple, cheerful environment.

The time you spend lovingly thinking about your baby while you are preparing his or her room will leave a lasting impression there.

Just as each house has a distinctive aroma, people can leave lasting impressions given off by their thoughts, emotions, and attitudes. When you radiate love and joy while preparing the baby's room, it is kind of like painting the walls with love. This warm coating will be reflected back to those in the room, even when you are not in the room yourself. Thus, as you fix up your baby's room, you are preparing it physically, mentally, and spiritually for your newborn.

If you feel skeptical about what I am saying, think about some of the places you have visited. Most of us have experienced the feelings of instant comfort—a feeling of having been in a new place before—or instant discomfort—even feeling that you could not wait to escape—in the atmosphere of a room. Perhaps it is because you were responding to someone's "vibes"—or a personal imprint that was strong enough for you to sense, either consciously or on a subconscious level.

So, what has your preparation for childbirth accomplished? It is just like when you were in school and had to prepare for an exam. If you really studied, did your homework, and were well-prepared, you would walk into the test room with confidence, feeling comfortable, relaxed, and in control of the situation. It is a great feeling. Your preparation will enable you to have the best chance at a loving, calm, welcoming, and joyful atmosphere for the birth of your baby and will help you feel ready, in control, and in sync with nature during labor and delivery.

When Is It Time?

As you come to the end of your pregnancy and begin anxiously waiting (and by now desiring) initiation of labor, the big question comes up: "How do I know when it is time to go to the hospital?" Of course, you should discuss this with your obstetrician, since individual guidelines vary a little, as do particular circumstances. In general, there are three significant situations or occurrences that warrant action.

If one or more of these occur, go to the hospital to be evaluated. These are:

1) The onset of regular, recurring contractions less than ten minutes apart;

2) Any significant bright red blood or active bleeding; or

3) Suspected rupture of membranes with corresponding leakage of amniotic fluid.

If you feel uncertain, it is better to go in and be checked and sent home than to not go and find yourself later delivering on the way to the hospital! By this time, you should have a bag packed and ready and phone numbers handy to alert the "team" when the time comes.

Attempted Early Arrivals

Yes, sometimes babies do come early. Obviously, a baby that delivers too early is at greater risk. A minimum of thirty-six-weeks gestation is always desired, however, babies delivered earlier than that can do well.

If you should go into premature labor, immediately call your obstetrician and start talking to your baby. Your doctor will probably send you to the hospital for monitoring. Sometimes it is just false labor, or Braxton Hicks contractions, and they stop. If not, and if you are less than thirty-four weeks, your doctor may choose to take medical steps to stop your contractions. This may include injections, IV medication, or oral medications. Do not panic, ask your doctor for full details of all the options, possibilities, and risks. Often, the contractions can be stopped, and you can make it to your due date. However, you may have to restrict your activity level until then. Remember, your baby can use your love and encouragement at this time.

Late Arrivals

What happens if your pregnancy goes beyond your estimated due date? Post-term pregnancy is a frequent occurrence. But by the time the estimated due date arrives, two things have usually occurred. First, the mother is more than ready to deliver her baby. Second, the word "estimate" has long been forgotten, and the due date has become etched in everyone's mind. This is an important time for expectant fathers to be patient!

Most babies deliver between thirty-eight and forty-two weeks from the start of the mother's last menstrual period, with forty being the number calculated for the due date. There is some difference in opinion as to how long a baby can safely remain in the uterus. Obviously, a baby can not remain for a lengthy period of time past its due date since the placenta eventually "wears out."

Once the pregnancy reaches forty-one weeks (usually considered one week past due), most obstetricians start routine testing for fetal well-being. The most frequently used test is called a non-stress test (NST). This is done in the doctor's office or in the hospital's labor and delivery unit using a fetal monitor to record the fetal heart rate while the mother notes the fetal movements by pressing a button that marks the tracing. By looking at the recorded heart rate pattern, your obstetrician can evaluate fetal well-being.

If there is proper reactivity by the baby, meaning an acceleration of its heart rate, usually but not limited to fetal movements, then all is assumed well for up to one week. Of course, this is not a guarantee but a reassurance. If there is not appropriate reactivity, two other tests may be conducted. The first is called a "biophysical" profile. During an ultrasound, the physician evaluates and numerically rates several factors, such as amniotic fluid volume, fetal breathing movements, and others. If a good score is achieved, it somewhat overrides a questionable non-stress test, at least for a few days. Your physician will probably then repeat the non-stress test within a few days.

A second follow-up test that might be done is called an oxytocin challenge test (OCT). This test requires a stay in labor and delivery and involves an IV drip. The oxytocin in the IV fluid prompts contractions, and the fetal heart rate tracing is watched for any slowing. All three of these tests may be used at any time late in the pregnancy, before or after the due date, to determine fetal well-being.

Using these techniques, your obstetrician can determine whether to give the mother and child a chance to go into labor on their own or try to initiate labor. If the decision is made to induce labor, most of the time the mother is given a diluted Pitocin/oxytocin solution through an IV. I try to avoid this method, but at times, there is no choice. I would hope your obstetrician discusses with you the need and indications for suggesting the use of Pitocin, which is sometimes aided by other agents to initiate labor. Remember, you have the right to know about justifications, alternatives, and risk factors. And remember that if you have to be induced, it is not a failure. Your end goal is a good outcome— a healthy baby.

The end of your pregnancy is a good time to talk to your unborn child and lovingly encourage him or her to get on with it! Do not underestimate the power of persuasion. Call it coincidence if you want, but I have seen positive results following such instructions as, "You are in the wrong position for delivery, you need to reposition or turn," and "I will be out of town, so you need to come into this world before I leave or after I return," and even, "If the baby does not come soon, we will have to deliver it by cesarean." Think what you will, but it cannot hurt to talk to the baby, and there is absolutely no cost involved.

By now, at the end of your nine months of pregnancy, your confidence and eagerness should be at a high level. You and your team should have a pretty clear understanding of what is going to take place and how to remain in control of your birth experience. You should know your unborn child pretty well by now, and he or she should feel loved and welcomed.

Part III

Labor, Delivery, and Postnatal Care

8

Labor

Stay Positive and Work with Nature

The Onset of Labor

LABOR CAN BEGIN at any time and in a variety of ways. Contractions may suddenly begin, your water may break, or you may show streaks of blood. None of these should alarm you. If contractions begin, start timing them to see how closely and regularly they are occurring. If your water breaks, if you show any red blood, or when contractions are less than ten minutes apart, call your obstetrician and your support team, and head for the hospital.

Finally, the time has come! You have everything organized and ready to go, but the most important things to bring with you are your preparation, positive thinking, a loving attitude, confidence, joy, and enthusiasm! All else will follow.

When you arrive at the hospital, you will be evaluated by fetal and uterine monitoring and pelvic exams to see if you are in active labor.

Active labor is when the contractions cause the cervix to dilate. Once it has been determined that you are in active labor, you will be admitted to the hospital. If you did not notify your team members before you left for the hospital, give them a call once active labor has been confirmed.

Clerical and physical admitting procedures will vary from hospital to hospital and obstetrician to obstetrician, but they will generally include some or all of the following:

- Getting you into a bed.

- Checking your vital signs.

- Checking the baby's well-being by hooking you up to an electronic fetal monitor to measure and record both the baby's fetal heart rate or tracing (FHT) and your uterine contraction frequency and relative intensity. This usually involves abdominal instruments attached by an adhesive pad or a velcro strap around the abdomen.

- Giving you an enema.

- Inserting an intravenous line (IV).

- Shaving around the vagina (prep).

- Cutting off oral fluid or food intake.

When I was training, all of these steps were taken automatically, and in many hospitals, they still are. I now feel, however, that the way to approach these procedures is to individualize their application. To illustrate, for years now, with no ill effects, I have not routinely used an IV with uncomplicated pregnancies. In my practice, IVs are only used if the patient is high risk or to prevent dehydration if the patient's labor becomes extended. I do allow some fluids or ice chips to be taken orally during labor, and I rarely, if ever, use enemas. Continuous electronic fetal monitoring is not required for uncomplicated pregnancies. It tends to restrict the patient's movements. If clinically indicated, I will, of course, use it.

I try to give my laboring patients as much freedom as possible within the bounds of good obstetrics. My patients are not required to stay in bed. They can get up, walk around, use the whirlpool bath, and find their own comfortable positions.

Some obstetricians have a difficult time giving up some of their control to the patient. The key is to find the right balance of physician guidance, good obstetrics, and flexibility for the patient. Most patients still do not feel they have a right to speak up and make their requests known. In my experience, patients do not often make unsafe or medically unsound requests. In fact, more often, I find that patients tend to "nest" in the labor bed and must be encouraged to experiment and ambulate, change position, or use the whirlpool.

What Is Labor?

Labor, as the word implies, is hard work. There is no question about it! There are three stages of labor. The first stage begins with active labor and ends when the cervix is completely dilated. During the first stage of labor, the cervix (the lower part of the uterus containing the opening) is progressively thinned out , shortened, and dilated by contractions, which are triggered by hormones. Each contraction causes the uterus to tilt forward and downward, while the presenting part of the baby, hopefully the head (vertex), pushes against the cervix, which continues to dilate to approximately ten centimeters when the head begins to emerge. With each contraction, the uterus becomes slightly smaller, and the baby adjusts itself as it moves through the pelvis. By the way, the word contraction is not synonymous with the meaning of the word labor. You can be having definite contractions, but they may not be accomplishing any progressive changes in your cervix, which is the purpose of labor. Ironically, the medical definition of labor does not involve contractions. Try to convince the laboring mother of that!

The amniotic sac surrounding the baby may still be intact at the end of stage one. Without interference, the amniotic sac usually breaks early on or near the end of the first stage of labor. When the membranes rupture, this is usually a good stimulation for labor.

The second stage begins with full dilation and ends with the delivery of the baby. This is typically the pushing phase. The third stage of labor consists of the delivery of the placenta.

When you reach the hospital, you already may be dilated a few centimeters and thinning out. A good labor pattern consists of a firm contraction about every three to four minutes. A rate of about one centimeter of dilation per hour is a reasonable guideline during the active phase of labor, but hard-and-fast rules need not be rigidly applied. A good mix of sound obstetrics, available clinical data, common sense, clinical experience, well-developed intuition, and patient input should be taken into consideration.

If a good labor pattern is not achieved within a reasonable amount of time, Pitocin, a hormone used to induce labor, may be administered by IV drip. Pitocin is safe to use but takes away from the "naturalness" of the birth atmosphere because it requires an IV and closer monitoring.

What is a reasonable amount of time to establish a good labor pattern? There is no absolute answer to that question. It varies with each patient and the overall clinical situation at the time the decision is being made. The first stage of labor may be prolonged, but a woman cannot stay in labor indefinitely. Both she and the baby will fatigue and start showing abnormal clinical signs. Some books and physicians try to apply hard and fast rules, but this is not the best clinical approach.

So, if labor is stalled and Pitocin needs to be used, it should not be viewed as a failure. Keep a good, positive attitude. If labor progress fails, this usually leads to a cesarean delivery. Relatively speaking, Pitocin use is far less drastic than having a cesarean section. Thank goodness we have means such as Pitocin to help achieve a safe delivery! However, whether the patient's own hormones or Pitocin is used, the contractions experienced by the laboring mother are essentially the same. The often held idea that contractions are harder with Pitocin is not correct. A firm contraction is a firm contraction!

Your Birthing Room Survival Kit

Here is a selection of simple items you may wish to have on hand during labor and delivery.

- Music and player
- Chapstick or carmex
- Hard candy
- Spray waterbottle for misting mother's face
- Lotion for massage (vitamin E or moisturizer)

  A firm massage to the lower back and feet between contractions can help relieve the discomfort and relax mom.

  Look for massage oils or lotions containing pure essential oils, such as clary sage, rose, and ylang ylang

- Aromatherapy Room Freshener

  A few drops of lavender oil in a dish of water is an antiseptic room freshener and some women find the aroma soothing and uplifting. Be sure to use only pure essential oils, in order to receive the aromatherapy benefits. Try this at home to see if you enjoy the scent. If you prefer, try orange, eucalyptus, or sandalwood essential oils.

- Loaded camera and extra film
- Socks
- Extra T-shirts
- Comfort robe
- Baby book for foot prints

Coping with Contractions

No two labor experiences are equal, even for the same woman. As discussed in chapter 7, each woman's perception of a contraction is subjective and individual. While I strongly advocate mental, physical, and spiritual preparation, realistically, even the most thorough prenatal preparation does not necessarily result in a pain-free birth experience.

Because they anticipate the pain of labor, women often fight the process instead of working with it. The media and movies usually portray the laboring woman lying flat on her back, sweating, and writhing in pain. At the same time, we live in a society that considers pain unacceptable—a sign that something is very wrong. These images make it difficult for women to remember that in labor, contractions and their discomfort are what move the baby toward birth. It may be helpful to visualize what is happening during the contraction and give yourself and your baby encouragement, knowing that the contractions are bringing you both nearer to each other.

The objective method of measuring the strength or firmness of a contraction involves inserting a pressure measuring catheter into the uterine cavity once the membranes are ruptured. I use this method very rarely and only if absolutely necessary. The less objective, but most used method is the perception of a very experienced hand on the uterus during the contraction, categorizing it as mild, moderate, or firm. The physician can also gain insight to contraction strength by watching the relative height of the contraction tracing on the electronic monitor when the abdominal attachment is used.

The first few contractions may take you by surprise, but you will soon learn to recognize the signals that a new contraction is about to begin. This is where prenatal preparation can be very helpful in terms of being able to relax and meet each contraction. Fear often plays a part in amplifying pain, and since many women are not properly prepared for childbirth, they enter labor fearfully. Fear and pain are also not conducive to maintaining a positive, loving attitude during labor. Eliminating a great deal of the unknown by preparation will help eliminate a lot of fear.

Although labor is largely controlled by hormones, it is definitely affected by attitudes and emotions. Stress and tension can temporarily stall labor. A positive, cooperative attitude, even determination, can help to keep you going.

Several examples can help illustrate how attitudes, expectations, and preparation can affect labor and the perception of it. I know a very wise lady who had her children many years ago. Talking about her own birth experiences, she said, "I didn't really experience any real pain during my labors because nobody told me it was supposed to hurt!" On the other hand, the fearful, ill-prepared mother with little support can certainly suffer during labor. At the onset of each contraction, she will scream and yell and tense up in fear and pain. As a result, the progress of labor may slow or stall out. The focus on the pain causes the patient to loose all control. When this happens, often the best course is to relieve some of the pain medically. Stadol is the most commonly used pain medication. On administering Stadol, it is not uncommon for the laboring mother to relax and begin to make more rapid progress.

The first-time mother usually needs a lot of support and encouragement to get through the first stage of labor. For team members, I would simply say, NEVER underestimate the importance of letting the laboring mother know that she is loved and supported. I will never forget the comment one of the support team members made during the first water birth I was involved with. During a particularly difficult contraction, the patient remained in complete control and breathed through it. After, her husband hugged her, and she said, "That was a tough one!" Her team member then whispered to her, "That means he is getting closer and closer to your arms." Both the mother and I were quite moved by the comment.

A laboring mother can also support her unborn child during labor by talking to the baby and urging her baby to cooperate, while reassuring her child that all is well and that she is happily anticipating the baby's arrival. Please do not forget that the baby is an active participant in the labor process and is also making decisions. Your love, support, and encouragement are invaluable to the baby's decision making. Can this be proven? No. Can it hurt to try? No.

During the first stage of labor, I encourage women to get up. Remaining passive and lying in bed on your back can be the least desirable position in terms of comfort and labor progress. Between contractions, it is helpful to move around and vary your position. Experiment; try standing, walking, squatting, or whatever position seems right for you. When you remain upright, gravity can work with you to further the progress of labor. As labor progresses, you may find that different positions feel "right." Don't forget to breathe. Simply breathing naturally and rhythmically, blowing out softly during contractions can be helpful. Your partner can help you maintain this pattern.

As discussed in the previous chapter, the whirlpool bath, massage, and nerve stimulation are helpful, noninvasive techniques for managing labor pain. It surprises me that more women do not take advantage of the benefits of the whirlpool. Whether this is due to "the nesting instinct," modesty, or simply lack of information, I am not sure. I encourage my patients to use the whirlpool and am rather liberal with the patient's use. I often find that it is hard to convince the mother to get in the whirlpool, but once in, it is usually even harder to convince her to get back out!

There are studies that show the technical reasons why immersion in water is helpful during labor, but common sense will tell you that the massaging jets combined with the water's warmth and buoyancy will relieve and relax tense muscles and increase comfort. Remember, athletes use warm whirlpool therapy for sore, aching muscles also. Of course, complications or the use of the epidural catheter preclude use of the whirlpool.

You may also welcome a gentle massage between contractions to help you relax. Even a hand or foot massage can feel good and help keep your extremities warm. A cool hand or towel at the base of the neck or forehead helps some women, while the reassuring touch of her partner's hand may be all others need.

Usually, patients who have opted for underwater births (more on that in chapter 10) have also made use of massage therapists during labor. One mother was surprised that the therapist massaged her feet and ankles, rather than her back or abdomen, to ease her contractions. The nerve connection between the feet and uterus makes this possible.

Some women find the skills of a chiropractor very helpful in easing the common aches and pains experienced during pregnancy, possibly due to the physical stress and spinal realignment caused by increased body weight and changing body contours. In fact, one patient of mine even stopped by her chiropractor for an adjustment on the way to the hospital to deliver her third child! She barely made it to labor and delivery before she delivered, perhaps due in part to the treatment!

As previously stated, I regard childbirth as a family's domain and I am not a "purist" who looks down on the use of safe (for the mother and baby) anesthesia. About a quarter of my patients choose epidural anesthesia to cope with labor pain. I see nothing wrong with using epidural anesthesia if that is the patient's choice. It provides good relief, does not sedate the unborn child, allows the mother to push after complete dilation, allows the legs to move, and wears off fairly rapidly. Unfortunately, some people view the use of epidural anesthesia as a failure or a "cop out." Do not fall into that trap. Discuss the available options with your obstetrician, and make the choice that is right for you! Obviously, I do not allow the patient with an epidural catheter in place to get into the whirlpool, but, with an epidural, she does not need the whirlpool anyway.

Tracking the Progress of Labor

During the first stage of labor, pelvic exams are done periodically to measure the progress of the cervix dilation. We do not want the mother to push against the cervix, so she must wait to push until the cervix is fully dilated. Complete dilation occurs when the opening is as large as the head of the baby and you can no longer feel the edge of the cervical opening. This is considered to be achieved at ten centimeters.

The pelvic exam also determines how much the cervical wall has thinned (effacement, measured by percentage). When the edge of the cervix is very thin, usually less than an eighth of an inch, it is considered 100 percent effaced. The third part of the pelvic exam involves checking that the baby's head (the vertex) is coming first and how low the head is in the pelvis (station).

There is another important aspect of the pelvic exam that most physicians and nurses are not aware of. This is the effect of the physician's touch on the unborn child. When a pelvic exam is done after some cervical dilation has taken place, the "presenting" part of the baby is touched by the examining physician. The unborn child has inherent psychic senses that are sensitive to the emotions, feelings, and "vibrations" transmitted through touch. As someone who is entrusted with the care of my patients' babies, I try to convey love, warmth, reassurance, and welcoming in my touch and in my intention.

During labor and delivery, there should be open communication between the health care givers and the patient and family. I feel that at any time during labor when a major decision needs to be made, the patient and family must be included in the process. It is the physician's responsibility to present the problem and the treatment alternatives. But, the decision should be made by the physician and the family together.

Since the first stage of labor can be prolonged, you will need to conserve some energy for the second stage. While remaining mobile or upright actually helps stimulate labor, as time goes on, you will need to rest more between contractions. There are many positions that can provide comfort. Among them are lying on your back with your legs elevated, lying on your side with a pillow between your legs, and kneeling on the floor with your head and arms resting on a chair. If you try out several rest positions while you are near the end of pregnancy, you will have several to choose from during labor. As the laboring mother becomes tired, it is particularly important that she receives encouragement and reassurance from those she loves and trusts.

As a woman approaches complete dilation, her whole approach to her labor changes. She may experience more intense contractions or several contractions close together. She may also experience dramatic emotional swings. This can be a time of increased excitement, with the thought and encouragement that the end of labor is nearing and the baby is soon to arrive. Everyone now gears up for the sprint to the finish line.

The transition to the second stage of labor may not be clearly defined. You may suddenly feel the irrepressible urge to push, or you may experience a lull. If a transitional lull occurs, take advantage of the time to rest and give your baby encouragement. Again, love and reassurance from your partner or a loved one can help get you through this period. Laughter, when possible, works wonders, but some women prefer quiet concentration. You are almost there!

9

Delivery

A Gentle Greeting

Labor: The Second Stage

NOW WE APPROACH the time all have been working for—the moment of birth. All has gone well during the first stage of labor. The mother has worked with and controlled her contractions. She has enjoyed considerable freedom during labor and has experimented with several different positions and locations (in and out of bed, walking, whirlpool, etc.). She has also been helped by the loving support of her team.

Up to now the mother's uterus has done most of the work through contractions. Now is the time for the mother to take a more active role. Now is the time to push.

While contemplating this stage of labor, I was suddenly struck by a startling but simple question: "Why do we tell the patient who has just reached complete dilation of the cervix to immediately start pushing with each contraction?" Other than, "because that is the way it has always been taught," and possibly, "to speed up delivery," I cannot come up with a sound, logical reason other than time considerations. There has been long-held belief that delivery must be completed within two to three hours. In practice, such rules can lead to more problems than they solve and increase the number of cesarean deliveries performed. Instead of applying rigid rules, the physician's best approach is to evaluate the total clinical picture, involving both the mother and child, and act upon the current conditions, using his or her best clinical judgment.

Whether or not the mother starts to push immediately, the uterus continues to contract and push the baby down the birth canal. Eventually, the mother will reach the point when she must push—when she will not be able to keep herself from pushing.

This overwhelming urge to push is triggered by the baby's head pressing against the pelvic floor. This stimulates nerve endings to send a message to the pituitary gland, which, in turn, sends a hormonal message to the uterus. The mother may actually feel a surge of energy at this point, caused by the release of adrenaline. As the uterus contracts, the baby's head moves down through the birth canal. As the head approaches the delivery it rotates allowing the shoulders to follow after. As the mother pushes, it can help to picture this process as it occurs, seeing the baby's movement and realizing that the baby is soon to be in the mother's loving arms. It brings great joy!

In keeping with my basic philosophy of cooperating with Mother Nature, it seems more appropriate to let the patient work with the contractions and allow the patient to determine for herself when to push. Naturally, there are exceptions, but I present this example as an illustration of the many medical practices that are perpetuated without question or periodic review. Patience is often a great virtue in medicine. It is one of the most important principles that an obstetrician can learn, and it usually comes many years into one's practice.

Of course, I am not the first to have this revelation. In fact, soon after coming to my own realization, I found this method endorsed in a book entitled *Episiotomy and the Second Stage of Labor*, by Sheilah Kitzinger and Penny Simkin. Among other things, the authors draw the conclusion that allowing the mother to push as she feels necessary helps to avoid or reduce the need for episiotomy, as well as the occurrence of vaginal or perineal tears.

In this country, women tend to give birth in hospitals, lying on their backs with their legs or feet supported. This position makes it easier to assist the mother with the delivery. In developing countries where women give birth at home, they tend to use upright or semi-upright positions. Squatting is occasionally used here in the United States, and some birth practitioners believe this position makes it possible to enlist the help of gravity. Any involved patient who is willing to experiment with various positions may find a more desirable position for herself.

Direction during Delivery

When the urge to push becomes inescapable, direction from the obstetrician can be helpful in coordinating the effort. Often, everyone standing by the mother is excitedly barking out instructions as birth becomes imminent. At times, I have to remind the excited group that only one voice should be giving feedback to the mother so that her effort can remain focused.

Proper instruction is very important at the time of delivery, and the obstetrician sometimes needs to take command of the situation in order to best help the mother. The most common situation of counterproductive instruction arises from enthusiastic family and friends all contributing confusing and often contradictory directions. Since a gentle, controlled delivery is the objective, the obstetrician is best qualified to decide what action to take, based on close observation of the current delivery situation, and can best serve the mother and her emerging child. When delivery advice starts to come at the mother from all directions, I simply ask everyone to help with their quiet, loving support so that the patient can focus on my directions. I have always found this effective. The "team's" intention is to be helpful, but as excitement swells, they sometimes need to be directed. A joyful, loving but quiet atmosphere helps the mother to focus and allows the obstetrician to assist the mother with proper instruction and gentle delivery assistance. By properly following a gentle, stepwise, shoulder by shoulder delivery approach, vaginal lacerations can sometimes be avoided.

Another example involving direction during delivery occurs when a patient loses control of her birth experience and fights Mother Nature all the way. Often, such a patient has entered childbirth unprepared and fearful. If the patient loses control and cannot handle her contractions early in labor, epidural anesthesia is often the best solution and can turn the mother's whole attitude around to her labor. However, by delivery, some women who have held on during labor totally "lose it," often screaming and writhing with perceived pain, making the entire process of delivery difficult on themselves, mostly, but also stressful on the baby and all others present. In such cases, the obstetrician has to take the delivering mother in hand, if necessary, by yelling louder than she is and demanding that she calm down, regain control, and follow directions.

This may seem harsh or uncaring, but when it is done out of necessity and with positive intention, it is amazingly effective. Often, the mother will "snap back into it" and will cooperate with her obstetrician to achieve a calmer delivery. In such cases, I always hope that all involved realize the caring impulse and the usefulness of the actions taken. Usually, the dramatic improvement and positive outcome speak for themselves, and the joy of seeing the newborn leaves the difficulty behind. However, sometimes the patient, upon reflection, will later feel unhappy about her behavior during delivery. Some have even come to me to apologize. I assure such patients that there is no need to apologize and advise them to focus on the happy result instead. I offer this example as another illustration of the importance of holistic preparation for childbirth.

Episiotomy: Pros and Cons

With each push now, the labia open to reveal the baby's head. Rapid, explosive, or uncontrolled delivery is likely to result in tears or lacerations. These can be avoided or reduced if delivery can be controlled so that it is a gentle, progressive process. Techniques, such as "ironing out" the perineum, may help avoid episiotomy or tears. This technique is rather simple and can be performed easily. It involves using sterile olive oil for lubrication. The obstetrician inserts two index fingers into the base of the vaginal opening up to about the second knuckle. The obstetrician then pushes down on the vagina firmly while slowly moving the fingers apart, out toward the lateral walls of the vagina. This is repeated numerous times to help relax and thin out the opening of the vagina. Supporting the baby's head, as well as the mother's perineum (the area between the vaginal opening and the anus) during delivery, is also helpful.

The main purpose of an episiotomy is to enlarge the vaginal opening to avoid tears and lacerations. During delivery, the vaginal tissue is stretched to its limit and sometimes beyond. As a civil engineer, as well as an obstetrician, I understand the principle that if you stress or stretch a substance (here, the vaginal wall) past its "elastic limit," it does not return to its original shape or size. This can result in a vagina that is enlarged and cannot be restored to its prebirth size. Therefore, the appropriate use of episiotomy is to make more room for delivery and prevent as much stretching as possible.

Episiotomy is a routine part of many obstetricians' delivery technique. On the other hand, there are a fair number of birth advocates who are strongly opposed to episiotomy under any circumstances. My philosophy falls somewhere in the middle. I am not categorically opposed to episiotomy, and there are times when it is definitely indicated. However, I do not do them routinely. And, if I could be fairly certain that a mother would not have a major tear or irreversible stretching of the vagina or perineum, I would not see any need for the procedure.

One of the most crucial aspects of long-term postnatal recovery is the proper anatomical repair of the episiotomy or tears. Unfortunately, in many cases, due to the relative simplicity and frequent performance of this procedure, the importance of meticulous surgical repair to the vagina or perineum is not fully appreciated, even by some health professionals. Rushing through the procedure or lack of proper technique can result in an unsatisfactory repair.

As an example of what can ensue from a poorly done repair, I will relate the story of Janice, a patient with an unfortunate history. When Janice had her first child, some years back, she was given an inadequate episiotomy repair. When she became pregnant with her second child, her new physician examined her, told her she needed repair, and assured her it would be taken care of when she delivered. Several years later, she came to me with major symptoms—diarrhea, pain, painful intercourse, as well as significant hygiene problems in the vaginal area. She was in sad shape emotionally and physically. To correct her problems, I did a major surgical revision of her perineal area, anatomically, layer by layer, repairing any tear or episiotomy, even those extending to the rectum. After healing, Janice told me she felt like a new person without any of her former troubling and uncomfortable symptoms! It is very rewarding to help people like this.

In my opinion and experience, episiotomy repair is taken too lightly, principally because it is considered minor surgery, done repeatedly and, often, in the middle of the night. Unfortunately, as illustrated above, improper episiotomy repair can cause serious problems.

I feel fortunate that I was taught to do such repairs patiently and correctly, and I am proud to say that I have had only one that needed follow-up.

Again, like other "routine" obstetric procedures, episiotomy should be individualized. If it can be avoided, great. If not, I do not hesitate to use it. Certainly, a neat surgical cut or incision is much easier to repair than a major, shearing tear. When opening size is critical to a good outcome for the delivery and the well-being of the baby, I will perform one and follow-up with proper repair.

Natural Preparation and Recovery for the Perineum

Women can help avoid both episiotomy and vaginal or perineum tears during delivery by preparing that area of their body during the last trimester of pregnancy. This involves massaging the area from the vagina to the anus daily with a vegetable oil, such as olive oil, almond oil, or wheat-germ oil, which contains vitamin E, a natural antioxidant. Vitamin E oil from capsules can also be used. Prior to massaging, a woman should first wash her hands. Sitting in bed, leaning against a pillow, she should lubricate the entire area with oil, kneading and massaging gently for about five minutes. This daily massage helps to keep the area supple in order to avoid tearing during delivery. The massage may cause a slight stinging sensation, which is normal.

To help gently heal the perineum after a repair from episiotomy or tear, try an aromatherapy hip bath. Simply fill an ordinary tub or a baby bath with a few inches of warm water. Then add a few drops of pure lavender essential oil to the warm water, mix well, and sit in the bath. Lavender is an antiseptic and anti-inflammatory and is believed to promote cell growth. It also said to have a soothing and uplifting effect on your spirits.

Prolonged Delivery

Textbooks provide varying lengths of time in which the baby should be delivered—usually within two to three hours after complete dilation—but this is nothing more than a general guideline. If the clinical data—baby's heart rate, amniotic fluid, mother's vital signs, etc.—are all normal, I see no reason to give delivery a deadline.

Sometimes in these situations it is best to do nothing but closely observe the situation until there is adequate information to make an informed decision. This is consistent with the philosophy of taking the lead from Mother Nature. At times, physicians may allow themselves to be pressured by a patient or her family into intervening when it is not necessary. Since most physicians are trained to "do something," it is hard, at times, to be patient, observe, and do nothing. If this situation arises during your labor, do not expect or demand immediate action. Respect and appreciate the fact that your obstetrician has the courage to be patient when patience is appropriate. Naturally, the physician should explain the situation to help calm and reassure those involved.

In keeping with a holistic, mind/body/spirit approach, the use of visualization can be very effective during delivery. The pictures you created and rehearsed during pregnancy, images of a safe vaginal delivery and of being united with your beautiful, healthy baby, can be powerful aids during this time. When women are in the late stages of labor and seem to be having a little difficulty getting the baby delivered, I often suggest visualizing "pushing" the baby out. With a positive attitude, this technique can be very useful in bringing about the desired results.

The Use of Forceps

One of the most misunderstood aspects of obstetrics is the use of forceps. Forceps are an instrument the obstetrician can use to gently grasp the baby's head, helping to ease it out. Their use requires skill, knowledge, and experience, but they have their place. The key to using forceps is knowing when and where to apply them, knowing how and when to pull, knowing when not to pull, and knowing the proper application and removal techniques.

Certain generally accepted obstetric requirements must be met for the use of forceps. The mother must have an empty bladder, and the physician must know the position of the presenting part and have adequate episiotomy and anesthesia. If the use of forceps can prevent a cesarean delivery, or speed delivery for a baby in trouble, I will not hesitate to use them. However, they also have potential for misuse.

Improper use of forceps can result in vaginal and cervical tears or lacerations, injury to the bladder, or injury to the baby.

Discuss the use of forceps with you physician ahead of time. Also, ask about his or her policy regarding the presence of your support person if forceps are used. Some obstetricians will ask them to leave if forceps are used.

I would like to share an example of "mind over matter" involving the use of forceps. This is a situation I have seen often enough to accept its validity. Often a patient has reached complete dilation but has stalled out and seems unable to push the baby out. On a number of occasions, after waiting patiently for Nature to do her work, I have asked the nurse, within earshot of the patient, to bring me the forceps. Then, I slowly unwrap them in front of the mother, put the two halves together, rattle them a bit, and then put them down on the table. It is quite amazing how many patients quite quickly proceed to deliver without the use of forceps. Thank goodness for the unlimited power of the human mind!

Achieving a More Gentle Birth

If you think mothers go through a potentially stressful labor and delivery process, just imagine what this newcomer to our physical world must experience! Being squeezed out of the dark, warm, quiet, liquid environment of the uterus through a tight and narrow tunnel into a bright, loud, cool, totally new environment must be overwhelming! This is why every effort should be made to create a gentle physical and emotional experience for the baby to remember and be influenced by.

Whether or not you have prearranged the logistical factors that can contribute to a gentle birth setting—soothing music, soft lighting, team support, talking to the baby—the most important factor is a calm, loving, and joyful atmosphere in the birthing room. My experience shows that the most crucial factor contributing to a successful, non-traumatic birth is the emotional atmosphere surrounding all the participants in the pregnancy and birth experience: parents, family, friends, physicians, and nurses.

Of course, gentle, calming music in the labor room can be pleasurable to the mother, her family, and the newborn. I have put together a birthing room tape for parents who do not have their own. It contains soft, soothing music and nature sounds that many laboring mothers have told me were relaxing and therefore helpful in easing their labor. Sometimes, in everyone's excitement, voices become raised. I gently remind all present to keep their voices down in consideration of the baby. While I am not in favor of watching television, especially during the later stages of labor, I feel that it is downright inconsiderate to the incoming child to keep the television on during delivery. Even small things like this can have an influence on the baby and the general atmosphere.

I strongly recommend continuing to communicate with the child during delivery, reassuring him or her that all is well and letting the baby know what is going on. This can be done verbally or non-verbally. I am sure there is no need to tell you to greet the baby gently and lovingly. However, I will remind you to keep in mind that soft voices and slow, gentle handling and movements help to avoid disturbing the newborn with additional physical stimuli. Covering the baby immediately with a soft blanket helps to keep the newborn warm. At this point, after all, the baby has known nothing but constant body temperature for its first nine months.

Gentle birthing advocate Dr. Frederick Leboyer recommends placing the newborn in a bath of warm (body temperature) water immediately after birth. (For more on water birth, see chapter 10.) I have no objection to the practice, as long as the baby is kept warm before and after the bath, but I almost never do it. One reason is that my patients do not request it. The parents and family are usually so anxious to get their hands on the baby they have waited "so long" for, they will not tolerate delay! However, if a couple were to request a warm bath for their newborn, I would comply.

Out of consideration for the newborn, my birthing rooms are very dim, with only enough light to do what needs to be done. About the only light I use in the birthing room is a fiberoptic light on a stand that only produces a small column of light. I even turn that light away from the site of delivery before the baby's head is delivered. Sometimes the light level is raised a little for video recording, but newer cameras require very low levels of light, so this is of little concern.

Within a dimly lit environment, newborns will often open their eyes, sometimes even before delivery is complete. Observing these infants, it seems obvious that this is not a glassy stare into space but a searching, directed visual exploration.

Once the baby has been delivered, it is time to present the baby to the mother by laying him or her on the mother's abdomen and waiting arms.

Having a baby is a major event in most people's lives and, generally, one of the most joyful. Certainly, families that have been involved, supportive, and loving from the start always display positive, joyous reactions, and from my perspective, it is enjoyable and rewarding to be one of the participants. I will give you an example.

John and Cindy had tried for some time to get pregnant. They were overjoyed when I could finally confirm that they were pregnant. John, who came with Cindy during the the entire prenatal period, was attentive and supportive throughout labor. He worked through every contraction and push with Cindy. When their daughter finally arrived, they were elated. John cut the cord, and I placed the baby on Cindy's flattened tummy. Cindy wrapped her newborn up and pulled her close. John waited by her side until he was ready to burst, and finally, he requested his turn to hold their new arrival. He initially held her as if she were going to break, but he soon became comfortable holding her.

The time this couple invested in their preparation paid off in the gentle, loving, joyous atmosphere that pervaded the delivery room.

I would like to share a more unusual example of a wonderful family delivery. Kevin and Lisa were both very involved in the pregnancy and came together to most of their prenatal visits. Occasionally, if Kevin could not make it, another member of the family—a sister, aunt, or mother —would always come in his place. I knew this couple wanted a "family delivery," but when I entered the birthing room, it looked as if the whole community had come to join the "party." All of the female members of both sides of the family were there, along with some of their male counterparts and several children. At one time, I counted fourteen people in the large birthing room, where the atmosphere was festive but under control. The level of attention given to the laboring mother varied from person to person, but all behaved well, contributing their loving support. Lisa did not seem to mind the crowd, although most couples would prefer more privacy. Near delivery, the number of visitors dwindled to a few close women. Kevin remained at Lisa's side throughout the delivery and was thrilled, after some coaxing, to cut the cord. The awaiting crowd cheered the announcement: "It's a boy!" Over time, all filed in to get their turn to hold or welcome the baby into the family. The baby seemed to enjoy all the attention. Because we kept the lights very dim, he looked around at the gathered family and barely whimpered.

Postpartum: The Third Stage

The final stage of labor starts when the baby is born and ends with the delivery of the placenta. This usually only takes a few minutes. After delivery, the uterus starts to retract. At the same time, the placenta begins to detach itself from the uterus, and the veins in the uterine wall seal off, so that the loss of blood is usually small and often contained within the placenta. After the placenta is expelled, the uterus contracts further, and the cervix begins to close. After the placenta is delivered, I examine the mother and do any necessary repairs.

Now that the baby has been delivered, welcomed by the parents, and wrapped in a warm blanket, and before the placenta is delivered, it is time to cut the cord. First, I clamp the cord, which, by this time, is no longer pulsating. Then, I ask the father if he would like to cut it. Most fathers I have worked with have been eager to cut the cord; some take a little coaxing; and a few simply refuse. There are no sensory nerves in the cord, so the baby does not feel the cord being cut. If the father is not willing, I offer the opportunity to other family members present.

The baby is now in mother's reassuring arms. Dad, along with other family and friends, is right by her side, touching and also holding the baby in turn. The baby usually has to make a short trip over to the warmer for the required foot prints, identification bands, etc. I always encourage the father to follow the infant to the warmer and stay by the baby's side. For fun, we often put a set of baby's prints on Dad's shirt. The law requires the administration of vitamin K and eye drops to prevent possible disease transmission from the mother. I do not like these to be done until the baby goes to the nursery, but the pediatrician usually controls those decisions.

Like other physicians, pediatricians feel more secure if babies are being watched by the nursery nurse. While nurses are certainly competent, they have to care for several babies at once, while a loving, watchful mother can devote her full attention to her newborn. I have found nothing wrong with babies staying with their mothers.

Who Cares for the Baby?

In most hospitals, once the baby is delivered, there is a "magical" four-hour period when the baby is moved to the nursery and comes under the care of the pediatrician. "Why," you might ask, "should a perfectly normal, healthy baby go to the nursery instead of staying with the parents?" That is a good question. I can only give the standard responses: "because that is the way it is done" or "to let the baby's temperature stabilize" or "to be watched more closely." I am sure any pediatrician would add other "good" and established reasons for newborns to spend those first few hours in the nursery. However, at this crucial bonding time, it seems a shame to see a baby lying alone in the warmer, not feeling the closeness and love of waiting parents. And if there are no medical complications, I know of no better or safer place for a newborn, during the first few hours after birth, than in the arms of loving parents. Newborns are certainly observed closely by their parents and could easily be checked periodically by a nurse.

If given a chance, I think we would find out that normal babies tend to thrive in the presence of loving parents. This has been shown in increased responsiveness, even in neonatal intensive care units. This is one area where parents need to advocate for themselves. There is nothing wrong with speaking up and letting your thoughts be known. Remember, it is often because you, the medical consumer, demands them that such changes in hospital procedure are adopted. Take some parental responsibility, and ask to keep your baby with you if he or she is doing well.

Even if your pediatrician requires the early nursery separation, do not forget about the remainder of the hospital stay! Most hospitals offer what is referred to as "rooming in." Hospital policies vary somewhat regarding whether the baby stays with the mother when she is sleeping. In any case, with "rooming in," the mother cares for the baby herself with some assistance from a nurse who instructs her regarding good infant care practices and techniques. "Rooming in" can be extremely beneficial to the continued bonding process between mother and child, and I heartily support it!

Nursing Your Newborn

Another important decision that mothers need to make no later than immediately after birth is whether or not to breast-feed. Of course, most mothers have made this decision early on in their pregnancy, but some are convinced of the benefits at the last moment. In fact, holding your baby to your breast soon after birth can help speed stage three by stimulating the hormones that cause the separation and expulsion of the placenta.

Most women's breasts produce milk spontaneously soon after birth. As the baby nurses, additional milk is generated. In other words, supplied upon demand. Nursing comes quite naturally to most women, but visualization and a positive attitude are always helpful. Occasionally, a woman may develop mastitis, inflammation of the breasts. This can occur when milk is not completely expressed or when a nipple becomes clogged, so be sure to wash nipples well after nursing.

As you would guess, I strongly recommend breast-feeding over infant formula. There is a great deal of literature confirming the health benefits of breast-feeding. Briefly, mother's milk is the most easily digestible and provides substances beneficial to the baby's immune system. Breast-feeding also establishes a special intimacy between mother and child.

Deciding whether or not to breast-feed, however, is a decision for each mother to make for herself. I would hope that those around the mother accept and support her decision either way. Taking a holistic view of the mother, I would rather see her happily and comfortably bottle feeding her baby than breast-feeding only because she feels she must in order to please others, while quietly resenting it herself. It is important for your baby to feel relaxed and comfortable while he or she is feeding; part of that is feeling your ease and comfort.

Infant Massage

When newborns come into the world, they must adjust to a whole new set of physical conditions. A good way to start teaching the newborn about his or her own body, as well as the comfort of loving, soothing touch, is through infant massage. When I have offered classes in infant massage, presented by a licensed massage therapist, I have noticed that not only do the babies benefit, but the parents do, too! These benefits include getting to know where and how the baby likes to be touched, while also learning a wonderful technique to help calm your child. The combination of learned massage techniques and a calm, loving voice does wonders for an upset baby's disposition. There are a number of books and videotapes available on infant massage. Also, check with a local massage therapist. Once you have learned infant massage, apply it during different situations: at nap time, when the baby is calm and alert, or when the baby is cranky. Avoid the mistake of applying the technique only when the baby cries. This will only end up encouraging your baby to cry for this physical pleasure. Infant massage has also been shown to be an effective treatment for colic. I urge parents to look into learning infant massage since it is so beneficial.

When Complications Arise

Like anything else in life, birth can have its imperfections. Sometimes they can be anticipated, and at other times, they occur suddenly and unexpectedly. Complications or high risk factors can develop before pregnancy, during pregnancy, or at the time of, or after, birth. Because all in the birthing room can be routine one minute and in crisis the next, the obstetrician must be prepared to respond appropriately and calmly. Fortunately, as a physician, most complications I have come up against have had happy outcomes. However, my personal experience has been less fortunate.

My own experience with a major birth complication started long before I became an obstetrician and was one of a number of factors that led me to become one. My second son was born with an unsuspected, major birth defect called spina bifida. He underwent his first surgery at six hours of age. Over the next twenty years, he underwent over twenty-five more. Because of my personal experience, I have a pretty clear idea of what other families go through when birth complications occur. During the years of surgeries my son went through, I learned a lot and became stronger inside. I accepted the situation and did what needed to be done.

Naturally, when complications do occur, excellent medical care is essential, and you need to trust the judgment of your obstetrician. There are all kinds of emergency situations that can occur. Some require split-second decisions and actions. In such cases, your obstetrician may not be able to fill you in as much as he or she would like. There will be time for that later. Again, approach the situation holistically; do not underestimate the power of positive thinking, prayer, and love.

It is especially important to enlist your baby's cooperation during these critical times by reassuring him or her of your love and support, no matter what the outcome. Hold and care for your sick infant as much as you are medically allowed. It has been demonstrated over and over again that sick or premature babies do better in neonatal intensive care units when they are held, talked to, rocked, and played gentle, calming music.

Of course, all this effort will not guarantee perfect health or complete healing. But, if you see that your baby gets good medical care and give your love and support fully, you will know that you have done everything you can for your child.

Many complications, however, do have happy outcomes. I would like to close this chapter with a story that may provide some insight to how the combined power of good obstetrics, time proven intuition, and love can sometimes avert a disaster at the time of birth.

This birth happened when I was on emergency room call. I received a page regarding a twenty-one-year-old mother of two who was expecting her third baby. She had little prenatal care and appeared near term when she came to the emergency room in labor with her membranes bulging, dilated four centimeters, and her cervix almost completely thinned out. The fetal tracing was normal.

I sent her to labor and delivery accompanied by her mother and sister. When I examined the patient, she was expressing pain and was dilated to six centimeters. I made the logical obstetric decision to rupture her membranes. That is when the first "red light" appeared. She had meconium-stained amniotic fluid. This usually indicates the baby has been stressed in some way and has passed stool into the amniotic fluid, staining it brownish-green. I immediately attached a scalp electrode to the baby's head to get a direct reading of the baby's heart rate. At first, the monitor strip showed a stable rate of about 145 beats per minute. Then, all of a sudden, the baby's heart rate dropped to about 40 beats per minute! This indicates a potentially life-threatening situation. As an obstetrician, I had to remain calm and draw on my years of training and experience to act instantly. At the same time, I was talking to the stressed, unborn child, sending love and reassurance.

I was encouraged by a number of positive factors present in this difficult situation. These were: the patient had had two previous vaginal deliveries; she was near complete dilation, due to pushing and some help from me; the baby's heart rate was slowly, but steadily, increasing; forceps were available, if needed; and my gut feeling and past experience told me this one was going to be okay.

On the negative side, the patient was crying and saying that she could not push. I could not give the patient any pain medication because it would further depress the baby since it would pass through the placental barrier from the mother's blood supply. I enlisted her mother's help to urge her daughter to push hard, while I worked on her cervix. The baby's heart rate was back up to an acceptable 120 beats per minute, and the head was visible and about ready to deliver. In such cases, you can never predict the outcome. With the patient's final pushes, I was overjoyed to deliver the head. As I did, I suctioned the baby to help clear the meconium that might have been sucked into the baby's lungs.

Upon delivering the head, I noted two loops of cord around the baby's neck. This was probably the major source of the baby's stress. I freed up the cord and completed the delivery. After delivery, I was thrilled to see that the baby was in excellent condition! Obviously, all present were happy and thankful for the great outcome. Babies do not always survive with two loops or even one loop around the neck!

I can only claim a small part of the credit for this happy outcome. As many of us in the medical community have learned, we have our limits. Did my loving thoughts and prayers help? I have seen many positive outcomes in the light of potential disaster, and I believe that communication with, and on behalf of, the unborn child is a great untapped resource that is available to anyone who chooses to believe in it!

10

Water Birth

A Special Experience

Seeking a Gentler Way

JUST AS I did not originally intend to help change the American birth experience, I never imagined I would become involved in and support the appropriate use of underwater birthing. As my work, my research, and my practice in obstetrics progressed, I began looking for more ways to make the birth experience as gentle and loving as possible.

Because my practice has always been within a traditional medical environment, I did not know or routinely encounter other physicians who were advocating a similar holistic approach to childbirth, combining accepted obstetrical principles with physical, mental, and spiritual preparation and gentle birthing practices. I admit for a while I felt quite alone. However, I did begin to encounter birthing advocates outside of the medical community, such as birthing facilitator Rima Star Cunningham. A dedicated advocate for world peace, she has assisted with many water births both here and abroad and gave the practice the ultimate endorsement by delivering her own children under water! Cunningham has also worked with dolphins, another intelligent species of air breathing mammals, and one with obvious expertise in water birth.

As I opened myself up to a world of ideas beyond the limits of traditional medicine, I began to meet or read about practitioners with interesting views. Europe and the former Soviet Union have always been ahead of the United States in gentle, loving, family-orchestrated childbirth. I have previously mentioned one of France's most prominent proponents of gentle birth, Frederick Leboyer, whose book, *Birth without Violence* had a tremendous impact on our consciousness of the baby's needs and experience during labor and delivery. Another Frenchman, Michel Odent, and Russian Igor Tjarkovsky are pioneers of the use of water with labor, delivery, and young babies, as well as advocates and practitioners of a gentle, mother-empowering, loving approach to childbirth. Odent, who originally trained as a surgeon, has been doing family-centered, informal, gentle water births for years, as has Tjarkovsky in Russia.

Gentle birth techniques had been practiced long before modern times. In his book, *Entering the World*, Michel Odent notes that a fourteenth-century monk, Bartholomew, believed that a newborn baby needs warm, muted darkness. Odent also mentions Hippocrates' belief that the unborn child takes an active role in its own birth. I have had the pleasure of meeting Michel Odent on several occasions and was honored by his attendance during a presentation I made on combining medical and spiritual principles during pregnancy and birth. This gentle and dedicated man deserves a lot of credit for demonstrating the benefits of nontraditional and gentle birthing practices.

Since my involvement with water births began, I have also had the pleasure of meeting Elizabeth Noble, a physical therapist whose husband happens to be an obstetrician. She has written a number of books and produced a video of her own underwater delivery. Barbara Harper, a dedicated holistic nurse and the founder of Global Maternal/Child Health Association, has an excellent book and video entitled, *Gentle Birth Choices*. I am sure there are many, many other loving and dedicated people all over the country who are helping to create positive changes in American birthing practices.

Before I proceed with the advantages of water births and a couple of waterbirth stories, I would like to restate that each couple's pregnancy and delivery should be individualized to suit their desires. One reason I wrote this book is to let people know that there are many ways to have a gentle, loving, and satisfying birth experience! Underwater birth is one way, but, at this point, it is still almost unheard of, particularly in the United States. In fact, it takes great dedication and persistence to arrange it, prepare for it, and achieve it! I am not advocating that all women should deliver under water, but when appropriate protocol is followed, delivery in a warm-water-filled tub is a safe method of birth and should be available to those who seek it.

The Advantages of Water Birth

For those willing to make the extra effort to pursue a water birth, warm-water immersion during labor and delivery has several benefits. According to water birth proponent, researcher, and practitioner Michael Rosenthal, M.D., these include decreased blood pressure and, greater muscular relaxation, thus less anxiety and lowered perception of pain. These factors allow the mother to work in harmony with Nature to achieve a more controlled, less painful, and gentler birth. Dr. Rosenthal also suggests that the more upright position assumed during water birth (versus the traditional recumbent posture in bed) promotes uterine blood flow and distribution, thus decreasing labor pain.

In his book, *Water Babies*, documenting the work of Russian water birth pioneer Igor Tjarkovsky, author Erik Sidenbladh comments that the buoyancy of water has a protective effect on both the mother and baby, through insulation, cushioning, and endothermic secretion. He further claims that any oxygen-breathing animal not exposed to the force of gravity has a significant decrease in its oxygen requirement.

As discussed in chapter 6, a newborn is simultaneously exposed to the powerful stimuli of light, sound, breath, air temperature, and touch! Warm-water immersion insulates the newborn, keeps him or her warm, and decreases the number of dramatic physical stimuli the baby experiences all at once. Water birth provides the newborn with a more gradual transition from the confined, liquid, prenatal environment to the new air environment.

For those adventurous spirits who choose to pursue a water birth, keep in mind that the details of the conduct and protocol may vary from those I describe, since all guidelines will be established by the obstetrician and the hospital where the birth takes place.

My First Water Birth

My involvement with water birth began in 1991 with an interested, enthusiastic couple, Pat and Ted, who wanted, in Pat's words, "the least traumatic birth possible." One day early on in the pregnancy, they told me that they were interested in pursuing a water birth. I initially told the couple that I would consider it and let them know. This was Pat's first pregnancy, and I had no direct experience with underwater birth. However, after thinking it over and delineating certain criteria, I decided to embark on my first water birth.

There are several reasons I agreed to this particular couple's request. First, I was impressed by their involvement and commitment to their unborn child. They both radiated love for their coming baby. More importantly, they had initiated the request, and they were willing to do their homework and take their share of the responsibility. I was also excited to be a part of a near non-intervention labor and birth technique, and I knew such an excellent opportunity would not arise often.

I explained to the couple that we would need some insight and guidance on how to proceed with plans and protocol, which, after all, would have to be written and approved by the hospital's executive committee. Coincidentally, the August 1991 issue of a respected medical journal, *The Female Patient*, featured a cover story by Dr. Michael Rosenthal about his experiences as the chairman of the birthing center in Upland, California, where 679 water births were conducted from 1985 to 1990. The article boldly proclaimed that warm-water immersion during labor and delivery had moved from a fad to an accepted procedure in some facilities.

Since I had previously written a protocol for the use of the whirlpool bath during labor, I was able to formulate a protocol to present to the hospital administration, along with the stated advantages and outcome information from Dr. Rosenthal's research. Since, over the years, I felt I had proven myself in the hospital, and I had a mutually respectful relationship with the hospital administrator, I felt we had a good chance to "pull it off." I spent a lot of time preparing for the event with Pat and Ted, discussing how we wanted to proceed, reading books, and watching videos I made available to the couple. The couple wanted "the comfort of a home birth and the security of a hospital setting."

Later in the pregnancy, Pat requested that her husband deliver the baby himself. This was the only request I denied because I believed it would not be safe. However, I agreed to all of the following (assuming all went well and no signs of complications occurred): no intravenous line (IV), no invasive or continuous fetal monitoring, minimal pelvic examinations, no medication unless requested, freedom to move around and labor in any position or location desired, clear juices during labor, gentle birth procedures and atmosphere, family and friends in attendance, Ted's full involvement, no episiotomy, video and still photography, and a few other details. In other words, it would be a non-intervention labor and delivery. We obviously agreed to follow safe obstetric practices at all times. I would be on hand to assist, evaluate, and intervene if complications should occur. Since we were in a hospital setting, I had to have the option of resorting to whatever means were necessary to insure a good outcome.

I also made sure the necessary supplies, equipment, and personnel were available. We chose a six-foot, round Rubbermaid agricultural tub, about thirty inches deep, as well as some garden hose and a pump and valve to drain the tank. Low-tech all the way! My office nurse, a spiritual and dedicated woman who was previously a labor and delivery nurse, assisted along with a hand-picked hospital labor and delivery nurse. They also prepared for this "first" with Ted and Pat. We even had a walk-through in Labor and Delivery with the nurses and photographer on the team. To avoid premature refusals or hassles from the traditional-thinking medical staff, I swore everyone to secrecy until near the expected delivery date.

Finally, about two weeks prior to delivery, we scheduled a meeting with the hospital administration. The administrator had guessed what our plans were, and she was willing to work with us. I was a little surprised to receive the two committee approvals I needed relatively easily. We were set to go! Because of their thorough preparation, Pat felt confident in herself and her body, and Ted was her most ardent supporter. The attitude, commitment, and efforts of all involved left me with no doubt that we would have a beautiful, uncomplicated water birth. We all felt we were in harmony with one another, with Nature, and with the entire process. It appeared the infant would come a day or two past the due date, and all was looking good.

As predicted, Pat went into labor one day past her due date, and we rallied the medical team, family, friends, and photographer. Initially, the labor progressed slowly and steadily. Pat and Ted strolled the halls with several attendants in tow. She spent some time in bed and some time in the whirlpool. Ted even got in the whirlpool with her! We also used the talents of a massage therapist during her labor, which Pat found very helpful.

We placed the birthing tub in the middle of the room so we had ample area in which to move around and videotape. When Pat was completely dilated, we filled the tub. Ted had plenty of room to be in the tub with her, and he sat behind her, holding her during the delivery. When Pat felt the urge to push, she did. With some direction, her pushing became fairly effective. To help avoid any tears or lacerations, I used the "ironing out" technique (described in chapter 9) to relax and thin out the opening of the vagina. It worked well in the warm water without the use of oil, as the warmth helped to relax the floor of the vagina. As we neared delivery, I urged Pat to feel the baby's crowning head. Later Pat said, "Touching the baby's head before delivery gave me such a boost, knowing I would soon hold my baby." When the moment of delivery arrived, the nurse and I helped support Pat's perineum, and I gently assisted the baby out into the warm water.

The newborn was very calm. After a short time, I gently guided him into his mother and father's waiting hands and brought the baby's head out of the water. The baby calmly opened his eyes and lay on his mother's chest. His heart rate was good, and he started breathing on his own with no stimulation. It was quite a picture of serenity and at-oneness with the world. Pat breast-fed her newborn while still in the tub. Ted cut the cord, and the placenta was delivered in the tub. The labor and delivery could not have gone better! Our holistic preparation served us well, and our instincts could not have been more accurate.

Our water baby provided all involved with a valuable lesson. Besides providing us with a perfect birth experience, he also gave me an excellent refresher course on newborn awareness, attention, and recognition. About fifteen minutes or so after the birth, the family was still in the tub. Ted was holding the baby close to his face and talking to him. "The baby felt a little tense when he was transferred from his mother to me," Ted said, "but when I welcomed him and introduced myself, his eyes moved toward me and looked at me. When I told him I loved him, he grabbed my finger and relaxed into my arms. I knew then that Alex knew what was going on!" As I watched the baby closely, I could see his direct and intentional gaze. You could see the bonding, interest, and recognition in the baby's eyes and facial expression. The established, knowing and loving relationship that had existed for nine months was very apparent. Ted and Pat had talked to the baby constantly during the pregnancy, assuring him that all was well. Watching them with their newborn confirmed for me all I believed regarding the unborn child's, communication and consciousness. If you have the opportunity to observe a newborn with her or his loving parents, it will give you a boost and provide a lesson about the inner-self and non-verbal communication.

I also give the hospital administration and nursing staff credit for their support. They were involved and cooperative. I had asked the pediatrician to be present at delivery, since it was our first water birth. I give him credit for being open-minded, remaining calm, and following good, commonsense medicine. He watched the baby closely but allowed him to remain in the tub with Pat and Ted for quite some time. After the family finally got out of the tub, he checked the baby and informed us that, although he expected it to be a little low, the baby's temperature it was, in fact, perfectly normal.

The videotape of this labor and delivery became the basis for my underwater birth tape, the only one I know of that shows a water birth in a hospital setting. I am very pleased with the tape, as it illustrates how a prepared, loving, gentle, noninvasive birth can be safely achieved.

A Positive Influence

The next water birth I had the privilege to be a part of involved a physician and his wife. Ed and Mary heard about my hospital-based gentle birthing techniques when they were expecting their first child. We immediately "clicked" and found we shared many of the same ideas and philosophies. They had deep spiritual insights into their unborn child. We all felt bonded with the child long before his birth. The birth itself was essentially perfect—a rewarding and joyful experience for all present!

Fortunately, although I have not done many underwater births, all those I have been involved with had no complications and great outcomes. The use of warm-water immersion during labor and delivery has been shown to be beneficial and safe for many years. As indicated earlier, I do not recommend a warm-water birth for every family, but for certain couples, it can be a safe and special birth experience. The desire for a water birth should originate with the couple and should be undertaken only if the couple is properly motivated and willing to do their homework and share the responsibility.

Remember, preparation, education, communication with the unborn, love, and gentleness can be part of any birth, as I will further illustrate in the following chapter covering cesarean delivery. If all these factors converge with good obstetrics, then parents have done all that is possible to assure a positive outcome.

11

Cesarean Delivery

Insights and Options

An Indispensible Alternative

FOR THOSE WHO are not able to deliver vaginally, and in the case of a medical emergency, there is a surgical alternative—cesarean delivery. Although there is some controversy concerning the significant increase in the number of cesarean deliveries performed in the United States in recent years, we should remember that we are fortunate to have a safe operative method of delivery available for those situations when medical complications would otherwise result in the loss of the mother, the baby, or both.

Who Needs Cesarean Delivery?

As mentioned, cesarean delivery is necessary when it is impossible to deliver vaginally, or when serious medical complications occur. Situations in which vaginal delivery is not possible include when the placenta completely covers the opening of the cervix (placenta previa); when the baby is laying across the uterus (transverse lie); or when the mother's bony pelvis is much smaller than normal and the baby could not physically fit through the opening (cephalopelvic disproportion).

Medical emergencies include the placenta prematurely separating from the uterine wall causing serious hemorrhage (abruptio placenta), the umbilical cord coming out before the baby (prolapsed cord), or severe abnormalities in the fetal heart rate. Medical complications with the mother, such as severe preeclampsia (toxemia of pregnancy) or a diabetic crisis, may also necessitate a cesarean delivery. There are also a fair number of other less frequently occurring situations in which a cesarean delivery is indicated.

As soon as you learn that you may need to have a cesarean delivery, discuss the decision in detail with your obstetrician. For non-emergency cesareans, you should be given the basis for the recommendation, possible alternatives, and potential risk factors. Your obstetrician should be able to present this information in a manner and language you can understand. Remain a part of the decision-making process; do not abdicate your responsibility or your rights. I have had patients who, when asked the reason for their previous cesarean delivery, said they did not know! If you are puzzled, ask questions so you can make the decision that is best for you. Obviously, in the case of a life and death emergency, there will not be much time for lengthy discussion, but there is always time, even as emergency steps are being taken, to give you and your family an explanation for what is occurring

Remember, cesarean delivery is not a failure. If the appropriate justifications are met, cesarean delivery is an important and necessary alternative and an indispensable technique. Make sure you know what is going on and why a cesarean is recommended so everyone involved can continue to work together for the best outcome. Do not forget to let your baby know what is happening and to reassure him/her with your love and encouragement. This, I believe, will assure the unborn child's full cooperation and effort.

Emergency Situations

Cesarean delivery situations can be divided into two practical groups: emergency and non-emergency. The emergency group can be subdivided into "STAT," or life-threatening situations in which time is of the utmost importance, and lesser emergencies, when time is not quite as critical. Examples of the "STAT" cesarean include heavy, active bleeding from placental separation (abruptio placenta); the umbilical cord protruding from the vagina prior to delivery (prolapsed cord); and a dramatic plunge of the fetal heart rate without recovery to an acceptable rate and pattern. A lesser emergency would be a less dramatic deterioration of the fetal heart tracing.

In the case of the "STAT" emergency, there can only be one priority, and that must be the appropriate medical treatment to avoid severe injury or death. In these cases, the mother's support team can help by directing their supportive and loving thoughts to both mother and child. In most cases, "STAT" emergency situations have good results for both mother and baby.

Of course, a "STAT" emergency cesarean is usually unexpected. However, familiarizing yourself with what happens during a cesarean delivery by reading or, better yet, seeing a cesarean birth video will make the situation easier for you to understand and give you a more secure feeling, should the need arise.

Two types of anesthesia are used for cesarean surgeries. The most commonly used anesthesia is spinal anesthesia. The most frequently used spinal anesthesia is called an epidural. As discussed previously, epidural anesthesia provides a pain-free surgical delivery, while the mother remains awake. It wears off in approximately two hours. Another type of spinal anesthesia, called a "spinal" or "saddle block," takes less time to insert and to take effect. However, the patient does lose the use of her legs while under its influence, and there is a greater chance of a post-operative "spinal headache." In the hands of a competent anesthesiologist—and most are—spinal types of anesthesia are safe and reliable.

The second type of anesthesia used is "general" anesthesia. Because the patient is not conscious when general anesthesia is used, she misses the birth experience. The recovery is a little more difficult ,and nausea following the surgery is more common. Thus, this type of anesthesia is generally used only in emergency situations when the need is for a very rapid onset of anesthesia.

When You Know in Advance

There are a number of circumstances in which a woman will know ahead of time that she will need to delivery surgically. Examples are repeat cesarean (discussed later in this chapter), a very small, contracted pelvis, and a placenta located over the cervical opening. These usually non-emergency cesareans can be prepared for physically, emotionally, and spiritually in much the same way that women prepare for a vaginal delivery.

The conditions and atmosphere of a planned cesarean delivery also do not have to be dramatically different than a vaginal delivery. Of course, cesarean delivery is abdominal and surgical and requires a sterile operative field. But, the conditions can be accommodated to the newborn, and the atmosphere in the operating room can be as loving and joyful as in any birthing room.

I always prepare my non-emergency cesarean patients with a cesarean birthing video I produced, and I encourage all patients to watch both the vaginal and cesarean delivery tapes so that in the case of an emergency, they will have some understanding of the procedure. To supplement the videotapes, I discuss with each patient the indications, procedure, and potential risk factors that could lead to a cesarean delivery. Then, I encourage questions to be sure that the "unknowns" are removed and we are all thinking along the same lines. Otherwise, all expectant mothers are offered the same prenatal preparation and education.

A Gentle Cesarean Birth

During the operation, the patient is fully awake and knows what is going on but, thanks to the epidural, does not feel pain. It is certainly understandable when a woman feels apprehensive about undergoing major surgery while awake. Here is another area where preparation can help. With an epidural, the patient can sense motion, movement, and pressure, but not pain. It may help to visualize yourself feeling the physicians' movements without any pain or speak with other women who have had one. If you trust that it will not hurt, you will not misinterpret pressure or movement for pain. Once a woman realizes that there is no pain, she can relax and experience the actual delivery and first sounds of her baby. Because she is awake and alert, she does not miss any of the excitement of the moment of birth and the first glimpse of her baby.

I always encourage the dad to join in the birth experience, and I have heard a wide range of responses from enthusiasm to refusal. I let the father know that he has the option of seeing as much or as little of the surgery as he chooses. Part of the surgical drapes are pulled up over a bar in front of mother's face, so the dad can avoid seeing surgery if he chooses. If the father does not want to be in the operating room, I will give the patient the choice of having another loved one, such as her mother or a close, supportive friend with her. I have even, at times, allowed more than one person in the operating room. For one cesarean, a family approached me with the request that I allow their ten-year-old son in the operating room to observe. After talking to the parents and the boy, I decided to admit him. He was great—observant and interested!

Some fathers find the surgery very interesting and watch every detail. I remember one father who entered the operating room with great reluctance. But before I was very far into the surgery, he was staring over my shoulder, did not miss a stitch, and asked plenty of questions! On the other hand, more than one "macho" man has had to be helped up off the operating room floor!

Before the operation, I put my hand on the mother's abdomen and have a few reassuring and loving words with the baby, letting him or her know it will soon be born and that all is well. In an emergency, I will ask the child for cooperation and assistance. Dad is usually at the mother's side, sharing the experience and often holding her hand.

The atmosphere in the operating room can closely mimic the warm, loving, family-inclusive atmosphere of the birthing room. While most operating rooms tend to be very bright, noisy, and clinical during cesareans, mine are quite different. The only light during the procedure is the surgical lighting that focuses on the operative field. The rest of the room is darkened. Just before the actual delivery of the baby, the operative lights are turned away from the operating field so they will not shine directly at the baby. This eliminates subjecting the newborn to such an intense stimulus as bright lights. At the time of birth, the atmosphere is quiet. Calming instrumental music or sounds from nature are usually be played to greet the newborn. At the time of delivery, I always talk to the newborn and welcome the child into the world. Other members of the operative team also welcome the baby, and then the parents are given a moment to see and welcome their newborn. It is always a joy to see the reaction of the parents to the newborn. Tears of joy, broad smiles, anxious talk, and a burning desire to hold their baby are all common reactions. Often, the father will cradle the newborn near the mothers face so that the three of them can have a loving conversation.

After the baby is delivered and turned over to the pediatrician, I encourage the dad or another family member to accompany the baby to the warmer. Since the baby is used to dad's voice and his presence, it provides reassurance. Then dad can carry the baby back to mother, and they can physically see and touch each other, talk, and lovingly bond. This allows the mother to remain active in the birth of her child, even though she is delivering surgically.

As with a vaginal delivery, if there are no complications with the newborn, I see no reason why the baby cannot remain in the operating room with the parents and then go to the recovery room with them. When an epidural is used, the mother is awake and alert and may choose to put the baby to her breast or just cuddle. With additional medications injected through the epidural catheter, the mother can stay relatively pain free for some time and can enjoy her newborn. Then, just as with a vaginal delivery, the newborn is whisked off to the nursery for the next few hours, although I would prefer to see the baby stay with the family.

So, it is possible to create a unique, loving, gentle cesarean birth instead of one that is clinical and impersonal. When you approach your obstetrician to request some of the conditions described above, be diplomatic. You may be relieved to find a positive reception, but if not, ask for clear, understandable reasons for denial. It is your delivery, ask for what you want.

Why Are Cesareans on the Rise?

Twenty years ago, less than 10 percent of U.S. births were by cesarean deliveries. Ten years ago, the rate was up to between 10 and 15 percent. In the last ten years, the rate has shot up to as high as 25 percent at some hospitals. That adds up to a lot of surgical deliveries!

Why are there so many cesarean deliveries performed? One reason is repeat cesareans. Once a woman has had a cesarean delivery, she will tend to have a cesarean for all subsequent deliveries. This practice has come into question in recent years, and I will discuss it in depth later in this chapter.

Many people attribute the increase in cesareans to the advent of electronic fetal monitoring (EFM). When the fetal heart rate is watched continuously, any undesirable pattern tends to result in a cesarean delivery to end any stress to the baby caused by the pattern.

The current medicolegal climate in the United States is definitely a factor in the upswing of cesareans. If anything goes wrong with the outcome of a vaginal delivery, the first thing that the doctor hears is, "If you had done a cesarean, everything would have been okay!" Most people, particularly lawyers, seem to feel that a cesarean delivery is the answer to any problem occurring during labor and guarantees a healthy child. This kind of thinking is nonsense but has created pressure to move toward a cesarean delivery more quickly.

The vast array of antibiotics and improved surgical and anesthetic techniques and procedures have lead to far fewer complications during cesarean delivery, thus making it a safer procedure. Hospital stay and recovery time are both relatively short these days.

And finally, cesarean delivery has become more socially acceptable as a means of delivery and has even come to be viewed as a way to shorten and end a difficult labor.

Once a Cesarean, Always a Cesarean?

As mentioned earlier, the often held belief "once a cesarean, always a cesarean" has contributed to the upsurge in the number of surgical deliveries. However, medicine has moved more toward vaginal birth after cesarean (VBAC). In other words, more and more women who have previously had cesarean deliveries are attempting subsequent vaginal deliveries whether by choice or due to insurance guidelines. There are still a number of obstetricians who will not allow an attempted VBAC. If you have had a previous cesarean, ask your obstetrician what his or her policy is concerning vaginal deliveries, after cesarean. Because there is scarring on the uterus, it is possible that during active labor, the scar may tear or rupture causing severe and potentially life-threatening complications. However, recent studies have shown the risk to be less than 5 percent.

When considering VBAC, there are some restrictions and considerations that will determine whether you are a good candidate for the attempt. Criteria vary among institutions and obstetricians, but one consistent restriction is usually imposed on women who have had what is called a "classical cesarean," with a vertical incision in the uterus. This used to be the only way cesareans were performed, and they are still done in a few specific instances, such as when the baby is positioned across the uterus in a "transverse lie." Most cesareans done today are called "low transverse cervical cesarean," meaning that the uterine incision is very low in the uterus and horizontal. The upper part of the uterus is considerably thicker (ten times or more) than the lower area. The upper part is also the most active during labor contractions. This puts stress on this area where a vertical scar remains and would pose too much additional risk during a VBAC.

When I meet a new patient who is pregnant and has had a previous cesarean, I first ask her which mode of delivery she would prefer. Women should have the right to choose, if a choice is viable. If she says she would prefer to deliver by repeat cesarean, then I respect her choice and the discussion is over. I am sure the idea of a long labor with the possibility of still undergoing a cesarean delivery discourages many women from trying vaginal delivery again. On the other hand, I do not want to discourage any woman from attempting a VBAC if she is a good candidate and that is what she wants. If the patient says she would like to consider a vaginal delivery, I consider her specific circumstances and obstetric history and give her my opinion. There is nothing wrong with trying, and if you end up delivering again by cesarean, it should not be viewed as a failure.

In some large hospitals, particularly tax-supported county hospitals, and under some health insurance plans, patients do not have a choice and with few exceptions must attempt a VBAC, even though many women would rather not attempt one.

While the reason medical organizations push VBACs is to save money, the truth is that the VBAC patient may require a greater number of monitoring hours than a woman who has not previously had a cesarean. It is not uncommon for an obstetrician to use both an internal fetal heart rate monitor electrode (attached to the baby) and an internal contraction monitor with a VBAC. Both are inserted up into the uterus and definitely restrict the patient's mobility. Large studies done at teaching hospitals have shown that it is relatively safe to use both Pitocin augmentation and epidural anesthesia during the labor of a VBAC patient.

Like many ideas in medicine, there was an initial rush to encourage women to attempt a VBAC. More recently, there have been articles in the medical journals that suggest that the universal push for VBACs should be reconsidered.

As with any delivery, and perhaps even more so, the woman's attitude plays a key role in VBAC. Women who have previously had an unsuccessful vaginal delivery often fear or feel resigned to repeat cesareans. Such women can help overcome this fear by preparing themselves holistically—physically, mentally, emotionally, spiritually—thus changing their outlook from negative to positive. Remember, all births that result in healthy babies, whether from vaginal or cesarean deliveries, are successful. Preparation helps a woman face and handle situations and opportunities as they arise.

Can Cesareans Be Avoided or Prevented?

By combining experience with good obstetric practices and personal insight, I have been able to deliver healthy babies vaginally in situations where some obstetricians may have proceeded with a cesarean delivery.

For example, a common diagnosis for many cesareans done today is "failure to progress" (FTP). "Failure to progress" means that the patient has been in a good labor pattern, but her cervix has not dilated or thinned. Quite often, a patient will make initial progress and then stall later in her labor. It can be particularly frustrating when the patient nears complete dilation and then cannot bring the baby down to complete the delivery. After a period of time, if no progress is made, "failure to progress" is diagnosed and a cesarean delivery is performed. Another frequent reason for cesarean is "relative cephalopelvic disproportion" (CPD), which means that the pelvis seems to be of adequate physical size, but for some reason, the mother cannot seem to deliver the baby. This sometimes occurs with a large baby (sounds reasonable) but is not uncommon with a normal size baby. This is sometimes called "dysfunctional labor." In these two clinical situations, patient, close observation and good clinical judgment can sometimes avoid a cesarean delivery.

Why does a woman who starts her labor well become unable to complete the vaginal delivery? The causes are multilayered and often not physical. Fear, fatigue, discomfort, and lack of preparation often play a part. In my experience, these cases often occur with women who have been somewhat ambivalent toward their pregnancy and have done little in the way of preparation. I have had patients who begged for a cesarean delivery because their labor was painful and they wanted to "get it over with." I want to emphasize that cesarean delivery is a major surgical procedure, one that should only be undertaken with appropriate medical justification. Pain management is a separate issue and can be accomplished with far less drastic methods than cesarean delivery.

Once again, preparation, education, and a positive attitude can make a difference. Desire and determination help, too. Do not be afraid to evaluate your deepest feelings. Accept responsibility for yourself and your situation. That alone can help you build your self-confidence so you can adopt a "can do" attitude. A positive, loving, and determined couple who does their prenatal homework and preparation do not often face a stalled labor situation. Remember, where the mind goes, the body will follow.

Let me give you an example. A patient of mine, Martha, had dilated to about six centimeters and then stalled in her progress. She was having a hard time tolerating her contractions, and after some time without progress, she was losing control. To remedy the situation, I asked her if easing her discomfort would help her relax, regain control, and continue to progress. I could see a look of relief on her face! After reviewing her options, I agreed to an epidural and immediately called the anesthesiologist. In less than the fifteen minutes it took the anesthesiologist to reach the birthing room, Martha went from six to ten centimeters dilation and was ready to deliver!

Why could she do in fifteen minutes what she had not be able to do in hours? From what I saw, as soon as she knew relief was on the way, she relaxed—mentally and physically—and let Mother Nature complete her effort. Her mind-set changed and allowed her body to take the natural course. The anesthesiologist went home without having to do the epidural.

Obviously, this does not work in all stalled labor situations, but if the mother's mind-set can change, the situation can often be reversed. Some women may take offense at what I am saying. Do not misconstrue my intentions. I am not implying that women in stalled labor are not making a tremendous effort. What I am saying is that while the conscious mind is trying, the subconscious mind may, for some reason, be blocking that effort. By starting your preparation early and creating a positive, loving, and determined attitude, you can improve your subconscious programming, which will help you to stay in control and achieve your goal.

Two other factors I mentioned that contribute to the increased rate of cesarean—electronic fetal monitoring (EFM) and the current medicolegal climate—are related and can effect a delivery decision.

In the early 1980s, electronic fetal monitoring was heralded as a tool that would greatly decrease infant morbidity (complications or disability) and mortality (death). Specific significance was attached to variations or abnormalities on the tracing, and the term "fetal distress" was attached to certain patterns. Studies and texts were written on EFM, terms were created and modified, and rules and interpretations were defined.

As I became more experienced in interpreting EFM strips and seeing the end results, I realized that there are no absolute interpretations or rules you can apply to EFM to always come up with the same answer, the best clinical decision, or the best outcome. General interpretations can certainly be helpful. But you cannot just look at an EFM strip alone and tell exactly what is happening with the unborn child or exactly what should be done, except in the most ominous tracing patterns.

Most obstetricians, including myself, on seeing a significant deceleration on the fetal heart tracing, have rushed the mother to the operating room for a "STAT" cesarean, only to deliver a perfectly normal baby. On the other hand, most obstetricians have also delivered a baby with a normal EFM strip, only to discover unexpected complications. The longer EFMs have been used, the more physicians have learned to look at the whole clinical picture—mother's history and condition, labor stage and progress, baby's position and EFM tracing, patient's attitude and support, medications used, etc.—before making a decision, particularly when considering a cesarean for fetal well-being.

Today's obstetric literature reflects the opinion that an experienced obstetrics nurse listening intermittently to the fetal heart rate with a stethoscope is as good a gauge of fetal well-being as continuous EFM. It has also been recognized that EFM read-outs are not always as exacting and predictive as first thought, so they should be used as guidelines, not absolutes.

Let me share a scenario. An obstetric patient of mine will be in labor doing well when an abnormal heart rate (HR) pattern starts to show up on the monitor strip. (This is usually in the form of a deceleration or slowing of the fetal heart rate.) If I am not in labor and delivery, the nurse will report it to me, and I will come to evaluate the entire clinical situation. Sometimes small abnormalities will escalate, and sometimes an abnormality will appear briefly without recurring. After making my evaluation, I discuss the findings and their significance with the patient and her family. Whether the abnormalities occur early or late in the patient's labor is important. If the baby will soon deliver, unless the abnormality is severe, it is often best to continue with a vaginal delivery.

One obstetrician may feel a cesarean delivery is necessary, based on a number of abnormal readings, while another may opt to wait or deliver vaginally with similar findings. The importance of choosing an obstetrician whose approach and philosophy you trust and share once again comes to light in such situations.

You may be wondering where this connects with the medicolegal climate and how this information can be helpful to you. Because of the medicolegal pressure in medicine, particularly obstetrics, many obstetricians will respond more quickly to any irregularity in the EFM tracing with a cesarean delivery or a forceps delivery. The medicolegal crisis is, in part, due to the fact that patients, their families, and their lawyers tend to want to hold someone accountable when the outcome is not perfect. No human is without error, including physicians. One can only expect the obstetrician to practice good obstetrics and do his or her best. There are times everyone has done a good job and the outcome is still not perfect. It is not easy to accept such an outcome, but sometimes it must be accepted.

Remember, a cesarean can often have the same loving, family-inclusive atmosphere and gentle conditions as a vaginal delivery. Let your wishes be known. If you need a cesarean delivery, work with your obstetrician, your family, and your unborn child to make it a positive experience!

12

Postnatal Care

A New Life Begins

THE LONG PERIOD of pregnancy and the excitement of labor and delivery is over. Now it is time to take your newborn home. Before you do, stop for a moment and reflect on what has happened over the past nine months. Looking back over your pregnancy, I am sure you will find all of your efforts to insure family inclusion and your preparations for labor and delivery worthwhile and rewarding. And now you have been blessed by the outcome of your love and your loving, harmonious effort.

Your Body Is Changing: Postnatal Recovery

After birth—delivery of the baby, the placenta, and it surrounding fluid—your body begins the process of recovery. Over the next several days, your body will release the extra fluid in the tissues, and your blood volume will return to normal. Within six weeks, your uterus will return to its normal size. Your perineum may feel sensitive and uncomfortable, even if you did not tear or have an episiotomy. If you had an episiotomy or repairs from lacerations, be sure to follow your doctor's directions carefully. After nine months of stretching, your abdominal muscles will be slack after birth but should tighten up over time, even without special exercises. Unless your doctor has advised against it, you can resume exercising soon after giving birth if you work into it slowly and err on the side of moderation. A brisk walk or other low-impact aerobic exercise can actually help a new mother feel invigorated, but heavy lifting and overstretching should be avoided for several months.

Fatigue is probably the chief physical concern of most new mothers and fathers. As you feed your baby around the clock, your body's normal sleep pattern is disturbed, leaving you feeling tired. Try to use your time efficiently, do not overdo it, and be sure to rest when possible. With so much to do, new mothers, especially those who have other children, must be sensitive to their bodies or they run the risk of mental as well as physical exhaustion.

Postpartum Blues

While science is not clear on why it occurs, depression following childbirth has been recognized since Hippocrates. In its mildest form, commonly called "maternity blues" or "baby blues," the new mother will feel low, irritable, anxious, or confused; she may experience crying spells and mood swings, as well as sleep and appetite disturbances. These symptoms usually peak within three days to five day after delivery and typically last from twenty-four to seventy-two hours. The primary treatment for this mild and transient disorder is supportive care and reassurance that it will pass. A reassuring physician and a loving, patient husband and family can help the new mother weather the storm.

Postpartum depression can also take more serious forms and, unfortunately, often goes unrecognized. It occurs after 10 percent to 15 percent of all deliveries and is much higher in adolescent mothers. All women are at risk, but certain factors, such as a personal or family history of depression, poor marital relationship, a lack of social supports, and child care stresses, put a woman at increased risk. Symptoms of postpartum depression include feeling "down," loss of interest in usually pleasurable activities, changes in appetite or sleep, fatigue, feelings of worthlessness or guilt (especially in relation to motherhood), and excessive anxiety over the newborn's health.

Many women who experience postpartum depression are embarrassed about feeling low at a time when they are expected to feel elated, but anyone who experiences such feelings more than a couple of weeks after delivery should contact their obstetrician or primary care physician. Postpartum depression can be successfully treated with medications, psychotherapy, or a combination of both. Early identification and treatment are the keys to successful therapy.

As with all areas of pregnancy and birth, understanding the factors that put a woman at risk can help her recognize and deal with postpartum depression. If you or anyone in your family has experienced depression, be sure to talk to your physician early on in your pregnancy so that careful postpartum follow-up is planned.

In my practice, I have infrequently heard complaints of "baby blues" and very rarely encountered serious postpartum depression. I feel that if you enter pregnancy with initial intent and desire, and go through your pregnancy with a positive, loving, and involved attitude, the chance of having postpartum blues is minimized. If you do feel overwhelmed or depressed, however, be honest about your feelings, and discuss them with a loved one or a trusted adviser. Seek help if you feel you need it. In most cases, these feelings are temporary and will pass with good support, honest dialog, and patience.

Who Is This Child?

Looking at your baby, you see a helpless infant. Yet, within that tiny body is a complete person. The helplessness you see only pertains to the child's physical being. The development of the soul cannot be determined by physical standards. Like many others who work in the birthing field and have studied newborns, I believe that babies are more in the spiritual realm than the physical for some time after birth. Close observation of newborns has made me appreciate the level of their awareness, involvement, and intelligence. The clues are subtle, and if you do not believe they exist, you might discount them. But if you open your eyes and your heart, you can learn a lot about and from a newborn. I have noted that in my experience, loving, involved parents who enlist gentle birth techniques seem to produce tranquil, calm, aware babies.

While newborns have a strong spiritual connection, they are also complete innocents, blameless, and incapable of wrong-doing. These qualities of innocence, newness, and helplessness make an infant appealing to those who are responsible for his or her care. Without these qualities, newborns would receive less nurturing and, thus, less opportunity to bond and connect with other humans. We know that children who lack emotional nurturing will flounder, even if their physical needs are met. Even tiny newborns need as much emotional nurturing as physical care.

Getting Acquainted

Today, we hear a lot about bonding with your child at birth. But bonding with your child, as I have discussed throughout this book, does not begin at birth; it begins at conception if you are open to it! Your loving feelings, thoughts, and words help create this bond. Some people even believe that loving thoughts can draw a child to them at the moment of conception. This is not hard to accept if you believe that unborn and newborn babies are attuned to the attitudes and emotions around them. We all need to feel loved, safe, and appreciated. Sending these feelings out to your child continually reinforces the bond between you. So, bonding is an ongoing process that begins at conception and continues long after the homecoming.

Practice Gentle Child Care

Gentle birth can be extended to gentle child care. During the first six months after birth, your child will learn to accept and enjoy the touch of others and will begin to know who can be trusted and depended on. If, during these early months, the child is frequently held, cuddled, rocked, spoken and sung to, and surrounded by a stimulating environment and loving people, the child will adjust emotionally, as well as physically.

Mothers often derive great pleasure from breast-feeding, both from the shared intimacy with their baby and from nourishing their child by their own body. Mothers who either cannot or choose not to breast-feed their children should understand the importance of holding the child during feeding. Under no circumstances is it wise to prop a child up with a bottle in the early months of life. This develops a dependency upon the bottle and deprives the child of the necessary physical contact with the human body. Focus on the infant during feeding; watching, cuddling, and talking are all a part of this special time. The father may also share the pleasures of nurturing his child during bottle feedings. The child who is nurtured and fed by both parents will be able to get to know and appreciate their different personalities, textures, voices, and aromas. Starting from birth, it is advantageous for children to be exposed to both the male and female influences. Parents who feel comfortable with their own mix of male and female aspects will reject outdated and inappropriate gender roles.

I strongly recommend that parents not encourage their baby to cry for what is wanted. While this sounds impossible, it can be done by observing behavior and trying to anticipate or promptly meet your baby's needs. For instance, when your baby shows signs of restlessness during sleep, rather than waiting for the inevitable crying, begin to gently wake the child, pick up and cuddle him or her, change the diaper, and offer food. While it is often not possible to anticipate your baby's needs, the idea is to avoid setting up a pattern in which the baby must cry to receive what is needed. Remember, it is a tremendous shock to the infant to be in an environment where these needs are not being met automatically. By reasonably meeting your child's needs, he or she will learn to trust that their needs will continue to be reasonably met. When the baby's needs are fulfilled before anger and frustration build up, the baby will remain calmer.

A New Family Life

When the newborn arrives at home, a new phase of your life begins. If you are first-time parents, your lives will be totally altered in profound as well as superficial ways. Even those parents who are prepared for the changes often find the reality overwhelming. To begin with, your daily routine will now have to be tailored to the new arrival. Settling in at home can be exhausting for new parents. Having family members or friends lend a hand for the first couple of weeks can be a real boon. A prepared meal or a couple of hours of rest can be the best gifts a new mother can receive.

If there are other siblings in the house, you will need to exercise greater patience and manage your time more skillfully. Siblings will enjoy the newborn, too, if their needs for love and attention are fulfilled. Pay close attention to the new dynamics in the household when the newborn comes home, and make every effort to compensate for siblings' possible hurt feelings.

Who Takes Care of the Baby?

Unlike their parents who separated "breadwinning" and "child-rearing" tasks, most couples today both work outside the home. As various social forces have kept women in the work force even after having children, men have taken on a greater share of parenting and household responsibilities. When both partners share their mutual responsibilities and help one another, life is easier for all.

New mothers, naturally, want to spend as much time with their newborns as possible. Most employers give new mothers a period of leave, usually from several weeks to several months, to get settled with their babies. This enables the mother to spend time with her baby, establish new routines, set up child care arrangements, and return to work without excessive anxiety. Sometimes an extended period of leave can be taken without compensation but with job security. A few companies even recognize the wisdom of giving fathers some leave after the birth of a child. Employers who have instituted such family-friendly policies have usually reaped a big payoff in worker production and job satisfaction. I hope that family-friendly policies become more broadly instituted as they are in Scandinavia and some European countries.

Work is an area where parents need to take initiative to be certain that they have the best situation for their family. Examine the possibility of working more flexible hours, job sharing, working part-time, working at home, or telecommuting. If you can come up with a workable solution, you may find your employer reacting positively. Computers and telecommunication devices have broadened the possibilities for working at home. However, working at home with small children underfoot can have its own pitfalls. Consider your situation carefully, and try to visualize the way you would ideally like to rearrange your life. Knowing what you want is half the battle.

With both parents working, who takes care of the baby? New parents need to feel comfortable that their child is properly taken care of when they are at work. A number of employers have established on-premise child care facilities that keep children close by in case of emergency, enable parents to visit with their children during lunch hour, and ensure easier travel logistics for the family. Some families arrange for a family member to care for their child. And many families turn to both public and private day care options. These must be carefully researched and examined for your own peace of mind.

Of course, many mothers do stay at home and care for their children. In some families, the mother is the primary wage earner, while the father stays at home to care for the children. It is not rare anymore to see a father in the playground during the day! In other families, both parents work part-time or flexible hours and share the child care responsibilities. Any arrangement that makes you feel comfortable and is embraced by both parents will work for your family!

Communication is important in establishing priorities, responsibilities, and loving understanding in the home environment. Be honest with your feelings, and share your thoughts with your partner. Learn to listen. By listening to your partner and your children, you will avoid many of the problems that misunderstandings can cause. As in all things, a positive, loving attitude helps you stay on track.

Role Models

Bringing a new life into the world is a big responsibility and requires a great deal of love, effort, understanding, patience, and insight. As a parent, you can help your child reach his or her unique potential by teaching social, physical, and intellectual skills and modeling your moral values. For many parents, this comes as a natural continuation of their loving and informed approach to pregnancy and childbirth. For most of us, it takes constant effort.

Children bring us great joy, but they can also cause us sleepless nights, worry, and frustration. They make enormous demands on our time, attention, and pocketbook. Nothing thrusts a reluctant adult into the grownup world like having a child. One of the challenges and, often, rewards of parenthood is the opportunity it presents to be the best we can be, day by day. Parents' behavior and attitudes are a model for their children. Contrary to what we would sometimes like to believe, parental behavior is a more powerful influence on children than parental words of wisdom.

In Summary

In this book, I have tried to present conception, pregnancy, birth, and even family life from a holistic viewpoint, recognizing that the needs of the body, mind and spirit are inseparable and interconnected. The ideas presented in this book have been assimilated over years of research and experience, both in my practice of obstetrics and gynecology and my personal life. If I accomplish nothing more than opening your mind to new ideas, I have achieved my goal. My main focus has been the practical application of the spiritual theories and principles I have learned to everyday life and to my profession. I refuse to be a part of the problems I encounter; I choose, instead, to be part of their solution.

As you reflect on the messages and guidelines in this book, I hope you will look within yourself and reflect on creating a better you, as well as a better birth experience. If you do, and if you earnestly look for answers, you may be amazed by what you find. It starts with love, commitment, open-mindedness, and introspection—imagining your true desires and believing they can be fulfilled.

Ideally, all pregnancies would begin with a loving couple's desire for a child and feelings of readiness. This does not always occur, at least not consciously. But, all couples can try to educate themselves about pregnancy, examine their options, contemplate and determine their special desires, find a sympathetic obstetrician, and have an individualized, family-oriented, gentle birth, whether circumstances dictate a vaginal delivery or a cesarean delivery. Open your mind to your unborn child. Realize that your unborn child is more than a developing body, and begin to make the child an active part of your family and your life.

Remember that pregnancy is a normal part of human life, not an illness. This is your birth experience. Take responsibility for it, and create what you want! You are the consumers in the birth-assistance marketplace. When enough parents demand reasonable flexibility from physicians and hospitals, their demands will be met. You are the key to needed changes.

I hope I have offered some ideas to spark your curiosity, some helpful guidelines, advice, and references, and some encouragement to pursue your desires and speak up for yourself and your baby. Please share this book with your partner, friends, and family. Discuss the ideas, and find your own way.

In time, as more changes and improvements are made to the pregnancy and birth experience, I hope they will lead to a true understanding of the benefits of a broader, more inclusive birthing team. I feel that practitioners of other disciplines—such as massage therapy, chiropractic care, body movement and alignment, hypnotherapy, acupuncture, religious and spiritual guidance, nutrition, aromatherapy, developmental education, and others—could contribute to each couple's unique birth experience with the obstetrician serving as coordinator. My ultimate goal is to create a family-oriented birthing center where gentle birthing techniques would be the norm and parents would have a broad variety of disciplines available to them so that they could customize the experience for themselves, their family, and their new baby.

One final word. My approach to childbirth could be summed up in a single word: Love. Love is the ultimate tool for the ultimate birth experience. If you approach your life and birth experience with unconditional love, you will make an immeasurable contribution to your own growth, your child, and even to the world. I wish you a rich, joyful, and loving journey through your pregnancy, the miracle of birth, and beyond.

Bibliography

Bry, Adelaide. *Visualization, Directing the Movies of Your Mind*. New York: Harper & Row Perennial Library, 1979.

Chamberlain, David, Ph.D. *Babies Remember Birth*. New York: Ballantine Books, 1988.

Chamberlain, David, Ph.D. "Intelligence of Babies before Birth." Paper presented at the World Congress on Prenatal Education, Granada, Spain, 18 June 1993.

Chamberlain, David, Ph.D. "A Journey to Oms." *APPPAH Newsletter*, Winter 1996–97.

Church, Dawson. *Communing with the Spirit of Your Unborn Child: A Practical Guide to Intimate Communication with Your Unborn or Infant Child*. San Leandro, CA: Aslan Publishing, 1988.

Gawain, Shakti. Creative Visualization. New York: Bantam Books, 1982.

Harper, Barbara. *Gentle Birth Choices*. Rochester, VT: Inner Traditions, 1993.

Harper, Barbara. *Gentle Birth Choices*. Global Maternal/Child Health Assn. Videotape.

Hewitt, James. *The Complete Yoga Book*. New York: Schocken Books, 1977.

Jordan, Brigette. *Birth in Four Cultures: A Crosscultural Investigation of Childbirth in Yucatan, Holland, Sweden, and the United States*. 4th Ed. Prospect Heights, Ill.: Waveland Press, 1993.

Kitzinger, Sheila and Penny Simkin, Eds. *Episiotomy and the Second Stage of Labor*. Seattle: Pennypress, Inc., 1986.

Leboyer, Frederick. *Birth without Violence.* New York: Alfred A. Knopf, 1975.

Leopold, Kathryn A., M.D. and Lauren B. Zoschnick, M.D. "Postpartum Depression." *The Female Patient* 22, no. 8 (August 1997).

Lidell, Lucy, with Narayani and Giris Rabinovitch. *The Sivananda Companion to Yoga.* New York: Simon & Schuster, 1983.

Nilsson, Lennart. *A Child Is Born.* New York: Delacorte Press, 1978.

Odent, Michel. *Entering the World: The De-Medicalization of Childbirth.* New York: Marion Boyars, Inc., 1989.

Price, Shirley. *Aromatherapy for Common Ailments.* New York: Simon & Schuster, Fireside, 1991.

Ray, Sondra, R.N. *Ideal Birth.* Berkeley: Celestial Arts, 1985.

Sidenbladh, Erik. *Water Babies.* New York: St. Martin's Press, 1983.

Tisserand, Maggie. *Aromatherapy for Women: A Practical Guide to Essential Oils for Health and Beauty.* Rochester, NY: Healing Arts Press, 1985.

Tisserand, Robert B. *The Art of Aromatherapy: The Beautifying and Healing Properties of the Essential Oils of Flowers and Herbs.* Rochester, NY: Healing Arts Press, 1977.

Verny, Thomas, M.D. with John Kelly. *The Secret Life of the Unborn Child.* New York: Dell Publishing, 1981.

Wambach, Helen, Ph.D. *Life before Life.* New York: Bantam Books, 1979.

Index

About the Author

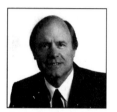

DR. RONALD COLE began his career as an engineer, graduating from the University of Missouri with both a bachelor's degree and master's degree in civil engineering. When Dr. Cole's second son was born with spina bifida, his earlier interest in medicine reemerged. He studied the causes of spina bifida, helped to develop special braces for spina bifida sufferers, and co-founded the Spina Bifida Association of America.

In 1973, he began his medical studies at the University of Missouri College of Medicine. During his residency and internship, he specialized in obstetrics and gynecology. In 1982, he opened a private practice in Baytown, Texas, just outside of Houston. He has counseled thousands of women in his practice and has delivered hundreds and hundreds of babies. He has also performed three underwater births.

As his practice grew, Dr. Cole came to realize the value of a positive, loving approach to childbirth and the intimate connection between mind, body and spirit in the conception, pregnancy and birthing process. He integrates this approach in his practice on a daily basis.

Dr. Cole's enthusiasm for life is not limited to newborns! He is a member of a world-record skydiving team, and his interests and hobbies include scuba diving, metaphysics, racquetball, four wheeling and ranching. Dr. Cole currently resides and practices obstetrics and gynecology in Baytown, Texas.